A PEOPLE FOR HIS NAME

By
Dr. M. A. Seiver

Copyright © 1989
DR. M. A. SEIVER   LAKELAND, FLORIDA

ISBN   0-931117-11-9

Cover Design - JOHN WALDON

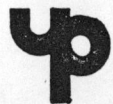

University Publishers
P. O. Box 3571
Chattanooga, Tennessee 37404

COMMENDATIONS

In this volume Dr. Seiver displays and examines the distinctive beliefs of Baptists against the backdrop of ecclesiastical history. He concludes, correctly, that while Baptists share individual items of their convictions with other Christians, the assembled mosaic of Baptist beliefs sets them apart as a distinct company.

Readers should find these pages interesting and informative. Baptists, in particular, will be grateful for this delineation of their distinctives and the reminder of their heritage.

G. Arthur Woolsey, D.D.
(From the introduction)

Thank you very much for the complimentary copy of your book, A PEOPLE FOR HIS NAME. I have read it with pleasure and profit. May God grant it the wide distribution it deserves. Every Baptist College should have one.

David Nettleton, D.D., Pastor
Fellowship Baptist Church, Lakeland, Florida
President, Faith Baptist Bible
College, Ankeny, Iowa 1966-1980

After carefully reviewing your manuscript, I am convinced you have done an excellent work.

James F. Dersham, D.D
Sunday School Consultant, Regular Baptist Press
Managing Editor, Regular Baptist Press 1979-1986

TABLE OF CONTENTS

Chapter	Title	Page
I	WHAT'S IN A NAME?	1
II	WHO SAID SO?	18
III	FAMILY AFFAIR	36
IV	SHALL WE GATHER AT THE RIVER?	54
V	ROCK-A-BYE-BABY	72
VI	UNHOLY MATRIMONY	89
VII	SWEET LAND OF LIBERTY	103
VIII	THE PROBLEM OF THE PENDULUM	119
IX	SAVED BY GRACE	135
X	PRIMITIVE BAPTISTS	152

A PEOPLE FOR HIS NAME...

A people for His Name, Oh, blessed folk!
They're called, from sin's dominion, to be free;
To be delivered from that awful yoke,
All thru' the blood of Christ upon the tree.

A people for His Name, Oh, blessed race!
They stand approved in Christ, their Federal Head;
Blameless, in love, before the Father's face,
Who, by His power, raised Him from the dead.

A people for His Name, Oh, blessed nation!
They're called to stand for truth against all wrong.
From earth they've heard no words of approbation,
But God has given them the victor's song.

A people for His Name, Oh, blessed people!
They're called, without the camp, to suffer sore.
No priestly class, or ornate nave, or lofty steeple
To furnish them with prestige, pomp, or power.

A people for His Name, Oh, blessed tribe!
They soon became "the martyr at the stake."
For their own life they offered no one bribe,
But chose to die like men for Jesus' sake.

A people for His Name, Oh, blessed seed!
The world unworthy of this people was.
They hid in dens and caves and there did bleed
For Jesus Christ, their one and only cause.

Now, these all have entered Heaven's glory;
In their hands the Nail Pierced Hands are clasped!
There, they all still sing redemption's story;
They've heard our Lord's "Well done, well done," at last.

From Heaven there comes a burst of acclamation;
From Heaven there comes a shout, "Praise to His Name!"
In Heaven they're singing songs of adoration
To Him who is through timeless time the same!

M. A. Seiver

Dedication:

To my maternal grandfather, Robert Marsh Anderson, now living in Glory; who, many years ago, introduced me to the biblical principles that are distinctively Baptist.

Introduction

Church history seems to indicate the emergence of two types of Christianity quite early in the church era. One writer has named these diverging streams "church type Christianity" and "sect type Christianity." The location of authority in religious matters was a major point of difference. Those of the "church type" held that authority concerning faith and practice resided in the church, while those among the sects were generally persuaded that the Scriptures alone provided the final word in these matters. There was also divergence in the category of worship, with the "church type" services tending to be formal and liturgical. Worship in "sect type" Christianity was ordinarily informal with an extensive participation of individual members.

In a similar fashion there appears to have been several currents moving in those times of religious and political upheaval commonly known as the Reformation. It was the "church type" of Christianity which was affected by the main thrust of the Reformation. This branch of the reformation movement has been called the "Magisterial Reformation." At approximately the same time there was a stirring among the Anabaptists and kindred spirits in some of the sects. This aspect of the Reformation has been given the name: "Radical Reformation." While both wings of the Reformation joined in proclaiming "solo Scriptura," there were voices in the radical section which proclaimed additional ideas which were destined to have a profound effect upon human history. Among these assertions were individual soul liberty, separation of church and state, and government with the consent of the governed.

It is superfluous to say that every major branch of professed Christianity is related in some fashion to these swirling events of church history. In this volume, Dr. Seiver displays and examines the distinctive beliefs of Baptists against the backdrop of ecclesiastical history. He concludes, correctly, that while Baptists share individual items of their convictions with other Christians, the assembled mosaic of Baptist beliefs sets them apart as a distinct company.

Readers should find these pages interesting and informative. Baptists, in particular, will be grateful for this delineation of their distinctives and the reminder of their heritage.

> G. Arthur Woolsey, D.D.
> President, Baptist Bible College
> of Pennsylvania (1960-1970)
>
> President, Spurgeon Baptist Bible
> College (1970-1979)

FOREWORD

Many histories of Baptists have been written; however, some of the best are quite wordy and exhaustive as well as exhausting. A number of books are also available on the subject of Baptist distinctives. Some of these are objectionable because they were written by authors who had an axe to grind. Others are written from a standpoint that is almost entirely denominational, making it difficult to get an overview of Baptists in general. Partly because of these reasons, many modern day Baptists have not taken the time, nor had the patience, to become knowledgeable about this people. Consequently, many are ignorant of the long history of Baptists and of the heritage we possess. Few realize the price that was paid by our predecessors who stood for the biblical distinctives of Baptists. Fewer still know how our distinctives came into being, or, what they are.

This work is not an attempt to provide a history of Baptists. It is an effort to tell of some of their struggles throughout their long existence, struggles caused by things for which they stood that set them at odds with others who followed a different path. It is an effort to show events in history that brought Baptist Distinctives to light and of the things suffered by Baptists because they stood firm.

Not only are these things shown, the effect of what others believed is demonstrated by the fruit they bore. Their errors are proved biblically and the right way is shown.

Throughout these pages we will identify the biblical distinctives of Baptists. These distinctives will be defended biblically. So, how our distinctives came into being and our biblical reasons for holding them will be the theme of many chapters.

But another subject will be treated also. Present day Baptists, in many instances, are showing themselves to be in danger of going against their own distinctives in practice. Ways in which this is being done will be shown and ways in which we can guard against this will be suggested.

As we proceed, it is hoped that we will come to a greater knowledge and appreciation of the importance of our biblical distinctives. It is hoped that the reader will see the importance of continuing to stand as those before us have stood. Only as we do this will we fight for the freedoms that are ours today because of those in the past who were willing to fight and die for them.

As much as is possible, I have tried to write objectively. What is written is pretty much a matter of history, i.e., that which actually happened. Past and present day beliefs and practices of Baptists will be stated, beliefs with which the reader might not agree. Please do not allow this to prejudice you against the overall thrust of this work.

I claim no originality for the material presented, only for its arrangement.

M. A. Seiver

CHAPTER I
WHAT'S IN A NAME ?

Primarily, names identify. We identify the person to whom we are referring by calling him by his name, such as Mr. Smith or Mr. Jones. But since many people have the same name (Mr. Smith and Mr. Jones are both good examples), another identifying mark is necessary. It would help make the identity more certain if we said, "Mr. Smith who lives on Elm Street." Another way would be to tell some physical characteristic or personality trait that distinguishes him from others who have the same name. When we do this, we are getting into the area of distinctives, that which distinguishes one person or thing from another.

Originally, names also described the person, at least in part, Those who study the origin of names say that many names distinguished one man from another by alluding to what he did in his vocation. Mr. Smith was possibly so called because he was a blacksmith. Frankly, I have no idea what Mr. Jones did. Perhaps Mr. Carpenter was — but you're 'way ahead of me, aren't you?

Scripture abounds in descriptions of the distinctives of individuals and groups. For instance, it is said of Barnabas, "For he was a good man, and full of the Holy Ghost and of faith: . . ." (Acts 11:24). Of the church at Jerusalem just after Pentecost we read,

> And they continued steadfastly in the apostles' doctrine and fellowship, and in breaking of bread, and in prayers. And fear came upon every soul: and many wonders and signs were done by the apostles. And all that believed were together, and had all things common; And sold their possessions and goods, and parted them to all men, as every man had need. And they, continuing daily with

one accord in the temple, and breaking bread from house to house, did eat their meat with gladness and singleness of heart, Praising God and having favour with all the people. And the Lord added to the church daily such as should be saved (Acts 2:42-47).

The disciples at Antioch must have displayed definite distinctives of being like Christ because they "...were called Christians first in Antioch" (Acts 11:26). Notice how well the name fits the distinctive. It was first given by the Gentiles who were not believers. It was possibly given in ridicule and used as a nickname for those who were followers of Jesus. But evidently they had seen that the disciples were, in their actions, like Christ, or Christlike, so they called them Christians. This name identified and described these believers.

Just as those mentioned above had certain characteristics that distinguished them, Baptists are characterized by certain distinctives. Their distinctives are principles that they have stood for and have been willing to live for and die for. They are beliefs that they hold dear because they believe them to be taught in the Word of God. They also hold these principles dear because they have to do with the individual's freedom in his approach to God in salvation, his liberty as he walks in the path of obedience to God, and his right of access as he seeks to worship God according to the dictates of his own conscience.

Now what about the name "Baptist?" So far we have only defined distinctives, but what does the name mean? Names distinguish a person, as we have seen. Just as some people were given a name that signified their vocation, Baptists were named for what they did. "Baptist" means "baptizer." Instead of saying, "John the Baptist" you could properly say, "John the Baptizer." So when they were nicknamed, for that is possibly how the name began, they were called "The Baptizers," i.e., "Baptists." This is the general meaning of the word, and for this reason some historians have referred to any group that baptized by immersion as Baptists. For instance, Seventh Day Adventists practice baptism by immersion. In the above sense they could be called Baptists. However, that is not the way we will use the word in this work.

There are several compound names that describe what certain groups practice with reference to baptism. They also tell what they believe about the ordinance. The following names are ones we will use a good deal hereafter, so we need to get acquainted with the meaning of each of them.

"Anabaptists" means "rebaptizers." In the Greek language "ana" means "again." We will see later that Baptists do not accept the baptism of those who were baptized as babies, baptized before they were saved, or baptized using the wrong mode, i.e., sprinkling, pouring, etc. They require them to be scripturally baptized before they are admitted to church membership. Those who opposed them called this rebaptism and called them "Rebaptizers" or Anabaptists."

"Pedobaptists" are those who believe in and practice infant baptism (Gr. Paidion, infant). Normally, their method is sprinkling or pouring, but that has nothing to do with the name. There are numerous references in church history to infants being baptized by immersion, sometimes by trine immersion. So "Pedobaptist" means one who baptizes babies, no matter what the method.

DISTINGUISHING THE DISTINCTIVES

There was a time when many who called themselves Baptists were well versed in their distinctives. Today, however, there are many who claim this name who are mostly, if not totally, ignorant of these principles that have distinguished Baptists from others in the past. They would be hard pressed to name those distinctives that have, historically, been held by those who have been recognized as Baptists.

Of course, most Baptists would name *Baptism by Immersion* as one of our distinctives; and it is one of them. However, many of them would not be able to give a good scriptural reason for doing it this way and fewer still would be able to give an understandable explanation of why our Baptist forebears were willing to die rather than do it any other way. Others, perhaps, would mention *Eternal Security*, not realizing that with the inordinate emphasis on man's part in salvation that is so much a part of modern evangelism, this doctrine is quite out of place. Further, while this doctrine is one that is held dear by the mainstream of Baptists, it is not a distinctive in the sense in which we will be thinking in this work. So what does constitute a distinctive?

DISTINCTIVES CONSIDERED NEGATIVELY

When I speak of Baptist distinctives, I do not mean that only Baptists hold them. To say that, today, would not be true. There have been times when this was quite true. However, a number of denominations that did not hold these truths in the past and were in fact, violently opposed to them, are now accepting and standing for at least some of them.

For instance, Leonard Verduin, who is of the reformed faith, has written an excellent book in which he deals with the struggles between the Anabaptists (our ancestors) and the Reformers. This struggle came about because the Anabaptists stood for many of the distinctives we will be thinking about; the Reformers did not. As a result, the Reformers violently persecuted the Anabaptists in an effort to stamp out those who held these truths, In the publishers blurb the following statement is noteworthy.

> The Anabaptists receive sympathetic treatment by the author, in part, he says, because "history has to a large extent demonstrated that they were in a large way right. Little by little, step by step, item by item, Protestantism has, at least in the New World, come to endorse the very emphases for which these men pioneered."[1]

Today, then, there are some who believe in and practice baptism by immersion; they do not baptize infants; they believe in separation of church and state. They hold some of our distinctives, but they do not call themselves Baptists and are actually far removed from what Baptists believe and practice in other areas. So, today, a Baptist distinctive is not something that is peculiar only to Baptists.

Second, I do not mean to imply that all who call themselves Baptists hold, or have held, all of the truths with which we shall deal. Different churches in different times would emphasize one distinctive above others and possibly almost to the exclusion of some of them. This could possibly be true because of conditions under which they were living and especially because of different foes they were facing. There are churches today, no doubt, that have strayed so far from what Baptists have believed and practiced through the years that true Baptists would not want to be associated with them. Yet they call themselves Baptists. Some of the groups in the past that have held to some Baptist principles have erred in other areas to such an extent that we would hesitate to be identified with them.

Third, a Baptist distinctive is not just a doctrine or doctrines that are held by Baptists today. For instance, the doctrine of *Eternal Security* that we noticed earlier, is one that Baptists hold, and have held dearly. However, we will not treat it as a distinctive since most of the Reformers also held it and it did not bring forth opposition from others as some we will consider did. What then, does constitute a Baptist distinctive?

DISTINCTIVES CONSIDERED POSITIVELY

First, Baptist distinctives are time honored. They have been held fairly consistently throughout the history of those who are considered to have been Baptists. Today, however, Baptists tend to be woefully ignorant of our history and heritage. Therefore, we tend to think of our distinctives as those things that have been in vogue among Baptists during the recent past, especially during our lifetime. I remember well, in the earlier years of my ministry, that in preaching on one occasion on Peter's sermon on the day of Pentecost, I remarked that the people cried out, "Men and brethren, what shall we do?" before Peter had a chance to give the invitation. I recently read a sermon in which the writer mentioned Jonathan Edwards' sermon, "Sinners in the Hands of an Angry God." He said that folks literally fell in the aisle as they were coming forward during the invitation. Both of us made the error of assuming that the present day invitation system had been in use through all of church history. Actually, the invitation system is of comparatively recent origin. It possibly began no more than one hundred and sixty years ago in the first quarter of the nineteenth century when Charles Grandison Finney began his practice of inviting seeking sinners to his "Anxious Seat" so they could be dealt with further in a personal way.[a]

I had also assumed that mention had been made of a pretribulation rapture during much of church history. Only gradually did I begin to discover that nothing definite was written about this subject until relatively recent times. It is now evident that it cannot be proved at this

---

[a]Dagg, J. L., D.D., *Manual of Theology and Church Order*. Harrisonburg, Va.: Gano Books. 1982. p 10

Sometime ago, I came across the following in a short autobiography in the above work. The event happened in late 1809 or early 1810. It shows that an invitation to come forward and profess faith in Jesus was given during a public service. This would have been about ten years before Finney and his "Anxious Seat." Dr. Dagg writes,

> Sometime afterward I was present at a meeting of the Long Branch church when invitation was given, to those who had hope in Christ, to come forward, and relate their experience. I felt strongly moved to accept the invitation, with others who presented themselves; but considerations, with the sufficiency of which I was not wholly satisfied, held me back....I left the meeting unhappy; and many an unhappy day of spiritual darkness and conflict followed, before I publicly professed Christ.

A PEOPLE FOR HIS NAME

time that the doctrine of a pre-tribulation rapture emerged, in written form, before the second quarter of the nineteenth century (around the year 1830).[b]

These facts are not meant as an attempt to show that the doctrine of a pre-tribulation rapture is wrong or that it is wrong to give an invitation at the close of an evangelistic sermon; they are simply statements that these practices and doctrines are relatively recent. However, novelty alone does not disqualify a doctrine, and just because the modern invitation system had not been used until a relatively recent date does not mean that it cannot be used profitably. It does help to nail down something that happened inwardly by declaring it outwardly. Someone has said, "Impression, without expression, leaves depression." These facts that we have given do demonstrate our tendency to assume antiquity when we are dealing with recency. Because of this, many practices and principles that are not time honored might be counted as Baptist distinctives when actually they are not.

---

[b] I recently read that a book has been discovered that predates this 1830 mention of a pre-trib rapture. The book is in the Oxford University Library in England. It was completed in 1790 and was written by Emmanuel Lacunza, a Jesuit priest from Chile. He wrote under an assumed name of Rabbi Juan Josafat Ben-Ezra and pretended to be a converted Jew. The name of the book is *The Coming of Messiah in Glory and Majesty*. Lacunza believed there would be a period of forty-five days between the two future comings of Jesus. He taught that God's judgment would be poured out upon the earth during that interval.

This book was first published in Spain in 1812. It was later translated into English by the Rev. Edward Irving and was published in London, England in 1827. This does seem to indicate that Irving had some knowledge of this teaching prior to 1827 since he would have read the book as he translated it; and, he probably read it quite thoroughly before he decided to translate it. This would have required quite a bit of time. It is quite possible, therefore, that there was a good deal of preaching about this subject, although nothing was written about it during the time he was reading and translating the book.

Also, since Lacunza did not complete the book until 1790, it is quite possible that he, and possibly others, were preaching what he set forth concerning the interval of time between the two future comings of Jesus.

A Baptist distinctive, then, is something that can be traced during the long history of Baptists. It has been held for a long enough time that it has become established, and it is definitely identified with them by those with whom they have to do.

Second, as we shall see throughout this work, Baptist distinctives have invariably been opposed by those who held doctrines and practices that were contrary to them. Not only were these truths opposed, those who stood for them were opposed also; and they suffered all manner of persecution rather than give up what they believed. Accounts of martyrdom are frequent in our history, as we shall see in later chapters.

Third, Baptist distinctives are principles that were formulated by Baptists as they searched the Scriptures. Therefore, they are the biblical distinctives of Baptists.

THE DISTINCTIVES DELINEATED

Having seen what constitutes a distinctive, we shall now proceed to present a prepared list of distinctives that we believe meet these criteria. As you consider these, notice that many of them are closely related to others so that they pretty much form a unit. This is especially noticeable when you consider their Bible basis and historical background during which they were made manifest by the actions of those who held them. Notice also that each of them stands independently by virtue of the first distinctive, which is our belief in the Bible as our only sufficient authority for faith and practice. Each of them stands on the authority of Scripture.

Second, notice that each of these distinctives is a belief, but these beliefs resulted in definite action. Everything our ancestors accepted caused them to reject something. All that they stood for caused them to stand against something.

Remember, these things that they rejected and stood against were things that were accepted by others. When a person rejects a thing that another accepts, not only is the thing rejected, the person is rejected also. At least, this is true in the mind of the rejected person. No wonder those with whom the Baptists disagreed considered them such a cantankerous lot. This has been true all along and will still be true today if we really stand. Now let's take a look at a summary of these truths.

First, Baptists accept the Bible as their only sufficient authority for faith and practice. Because of this they reject the authority of councils, creeds, tradition, and hierarchal utterances unless they agree with Scripture. If they do agree, their authority still depends on Scripture. This does not mean that Baptists do not value the decisions of councils and the creeds which they produced. They just reject them as a final authority and look only to Scripture. It is their supreme court of appeal.

Second, Baptists believe in a regenerate church membership. Only those who have been born again, regenerated, can be received into the membership of the church. Unsaved adults and infants are rejected. Adults must at least profess salvation, and in some cases they have been required to give a verbal testimony of their salvation experience and give evidence in their lives that they have been converted. Infants cannot be saved, nor do they need to be. Salvation is by grace, through faith, and an infant cannot exercise faith. They are safe, however, not because they are infants but because of God's grace.

Third, Baptists believe in baptism by immersion and of believers only. This alone constitutes biblical baptism. They reject those who have been sprinkled, etc. They must be baptized biblically. Because belief must precede baptism, they reject infant baptism. Further, they insist that those who went through the baptismal ceremony before they were saved must be baptized after they are saved. Otherwise, their's is not a biblical baptism. This has caused quite a furor among those who opposed the Baptists. They called it rebaptism, and Baptists suffered much persecution because of this practice. It is in the areas of infant baptism, baptism of believers only, and baptism by immersion that Baptists are singularly opposed by others to this day.

Fourth, Baptists believe in soul liberty or freedom of conscience. They do not believe that any civil or religious power has any right to dictate what they must believe in spiritual matters. Because of this belief, they have stood against a practice that has been used much during the history of the church. That practice came about when certain segments of the church used the civil powers to coerce individuals to believe their way. This will form an interesting part of our discussion in later chapters, and we shall see that it led to the belief in separation of church and state. It was by the union of civil and religious powers that the earth has been stained by the blood of martyrs and the air has been polluted by the stench of burning bodies as men were put to death in the most horrible ways because they refused to believe what someone else demanded they believe. This would not have been possible, to such an extent, without the cooperation of the civil government. It was against this black backdrop that many fled to the New World to escape religious persecution, and it is because of those who tenaciously held the principle of soul liberty that we in the United States enjoy religious freedom today.

Fifth, Baptists believe in an equal brotherhood of believers. They hold that all believers are priests and that each has direct access to God through Jesus Christ our mediator. They do not have to go through the preacher. Because of this belief, they reject any order of priests who could grant them access to God or deny such access. Since their access to God is through the one mediator, Jesus Christ, they do not believe it is necessary or proper to pray through Mary or some saint. They also deny any teaching about the Lord's Supper that requires the mediation of a priest to make it beneficial to them. This would require an unequal brotherhood and deny them soul liberty.

Further, their equal brotherhood belief based upon the teaching of Scripture leads them to govern themselves by a congregational form of government. They are not ruled by a board of elders or deacons. Nor do they allow any ecclesiastical power outside the local church to exercise control over them.

Sixth, Baptists believe in salvation by grace, through faith. The above-mentioned faith is personal faith. The one who is saved is the one who believes. This caused Baptists to reject proxy faith, or parents believing for their children. They also reject any system that makes necessary the intervention of a priest to convey salvation; and neither of the two ordinances, Baptism and the Lord's Supper, has any salvific value. These things separate Baptists from others by a vast distance .

Seventh, Baptists believe in maintaining the original order of the church. This is the primitive order, the way things ought to be done according to Scripture. No matter what kind of order has developed since Bible times, or if no order at all has been maintained, Scripture is still the manual of church order. Since this includes all of the distinctives, it is needless to say that much opposition and persecution have resulted. Maintaining this order has definitely set Baptists apart from many and has evoked a good deal of ridicule and differing opinions from others. They have, however, stood fairly consistently, even during recent days when Baptists seem to desire to "be like all the nations."

ROOTS

Numerous statements have been made so far implying that Baptists have been around for a long time. To what extent this is true and with what degree of continuity has set the stage for much controversy in the past and, to some degree, in the present, even among Baptists. In the nineteenth century the "Landmarker" controversy raged among Southern Baptists and in some areas, is still being fought today. At the center of this debate were several theories concerning the continuity of Baptists. Among these were:

(1) Church Succession, the belief that for a church to be a true church it must have grown out of a church that grew out of a church, etc., all the way back to the first Baptist church in New Testament times and,

(2) Baptismal Succession, the belief that for baptism to be valid you must be baptized by someone who was baptized by someone, etc., all the way back to the time of Jesus or even back to the baptism of John.

I have heard of one account of a Baptist church in the South that claims to be able to trace a succession all the way back to the time of Jesus. However, it is certain that very few people could verify their baptism by such a procedure, even if this church could prove an authentic succession. Church historian Thomas Armitage says, "Such evidence cannot be traced by any church on earth, and would be utterly worthless if it could, because the real legitimacy of Christianity must be found in the New Testament, and nowhere else."[2]

Further, if such a thing were possible it could easily lead to unwarranted pride and, possibly, to a popish stance that would contradict principles which are definitely based on the Bible. Baptists, with weighty arguments, have opposed the doctrine of papal succession; yet some of these same Baptists, attempting to build a doctrine of church succession, put themselves in danger of committing the same error. It is my position that the authenticity of a Baptist church does not depend upon its ancestry but upon its adherence to the teachings of the Word of God.

What has just been said is not an attempt to disprove succession. This might be a fact; proving it is another matter. Further, a succession of Baptist churches is not germane to our discussion here. Our authority is from Scripture, not from others in the past who held the same belief. At this point, however, it is important that we see the difference between succession and antiquity. Good says,

> A careful distinction needs to be made between antiquity and continuity. The first is agreed upon by Baptists, and they are fully supported by reliable historians from other churches. As to the second, there is a divergence of opinion.[3]

A PEOPLE FOR HIS NAME

He, therefore, concludes that antiquity is well established. Baptists are an ancient people.

The ways in which historians and other writers have come to the conclusion that Baptist churches have existed throughout the history of the church are very interesting. One does it by defining a New Testament church in the following way. He writes,

> ... Only two doctrines are essential to a New Testament church. Other doctrines are important, precious, but only two are essential to a New Testament church. They are the WAY OF SALVATION and the WAY OF BAPTISM[4] (Emphases are his).

According to him, a church that is right on these two things is a Baptist church, and he finds such churches all the way back to the apostles. It is evident that he believes that a New Testament church is a Baptist church.

Another gives three rules by which he determines the antiquity of Baptists. They are,

> (1) The existence of ancient records which give testimony to the practice of our principles in groups which carried on the gospel witness and maintained New Testament churches in all times dating back to the apostles.
> (2) The failure of historians to locate any specific time in post-apostolic history when the Baptists began.
> (3) The recognition among historians that ancient traditions are valid criteria for tracing origins.[5]

Both of these that we have just quoted are Baptists; one of them is a successionist but the other is not.

Leonard Verduin, our friend of the reformed faith and not a Baptist, shows that the Anabaptists were opposed and persecuted by the Reformers because of principles that had been held by certain groups in the church for at least the past twelve hundred years (344-1519). He writes,

> ... When Josef Beck set himself to edit a volume of original source materials, ...he deftly exscinded "a piece of church history extending from the year 344 to 1519" for the reason that it "had nothing at all, or very little, to do with the matter in hand." Surely this is arbitrary procedure. The people who wrote this early account - their own biography - were of the conviction that one must pay considerable attention to the events that lie between 344 and 1519 if one is to understand the origin and history of the people described....[6]

This gives evidence of his belief in the antiquity of churches holding the doctrinal principles of the Anabaptists, the forerunners of present day Baptists.

Briefly, we have noted the methods used by Baptists, non-Baptists, successionists, and non-successionists. Their conclusions are clearly similar; groups holding Baptist principles have been in existence since New Testament times. This is the reason Baptists are not Protestant. They were already in existence at the time of the Reformation and were holding the truths they had always held although they had a different name, Anabaptists. They did cooperate briefly with the Reformers, but soon discovered that they were not going far enough in the right direction. The Anabaptists did not believe the Reformers were willing to make a complete break with the Roman Catholic Church since they still retained, among other things, the Catholic errors of infant baptism and the State-Church, both of which were directly opposed to the principles of the Anabaptists. The Reformers became antagonistic toward them; and persecution by the Reformers was severe, as it had been at the hands of the Catholic Church. Because of this, they remained separate as they had been and continued standing for the truth as they had been standing. They did not have their beginning in the Reformation and they never were really a part of the Protestant movement. Therefore, they are not Protestant.

We must understand that no claim is made of a people who bore the Baptist name. This name can be traced back only a few hundred years, with the exception of John the Baptist. However, Baptist principles can be traced as they were practiced by groups that were known as Montanists, Novatians, Donatists, Paulicians, Waldenses, and the Anabaptists. It may be objected that these were not pure churches, and that they committed error in the matter of doctrine and in practice. We reply that there are no pure churches today; there never have been and there never will be. Some of the above did hold doctrine with which we would not agree. But they were also instrumental in formulating and establishing the principles we claim today as our distinctives. Some possibly held to all the distinctives, some to only a part of them. But they did hold principles that are distinctively Baptist.

A ROSE BY ANY OTHER NAME

Now what does all this mean to us? There is evidence that it does not mean much to many. In a recent religious survey it was discovered that most people do not choose the church they attend on the basis of doctrine, preaching, or denomination; but they choose it for the music, youth program, or social program. They do not choose their church because of what it stands for; they choose it because of what it offers them. This practice has not always been as prevalent as it is now. I remember hearing those of a past generation speak of choosing a church on the basis of how closely it aligned itself with the teachings of Scripture. There was a time when many became Baptists because they held their principles and teachings dear.

Today, it seems that many are Baptists because they were saved in a Baptist church and it was only logical that they remain there. They do not seem to know that there is any difference between Baptist churches and others. They refer to themselves as "Protestant" or at best "non-Catholic." They do not know why there is a difference. This would not be true if they were not ignorant of what Baptists have endured and stood for in the past. Someone has said, "He who ignores history is destined to repeat history." If we remain ignorant of our heritage and history we may find ourselves suffering some of the same things our ancestors suffered. A thorough knowledge of our distinctives that have come from the Word of God and have been tested and tempered in the crucible of persecution and suffering will help prevent this.

History reveals that those who have stood for our distinctives have been known by many different names, as we have just seen. Sometimes a group would stand for the truth and then succumb to error. But God was faithful to raise up another group with a different name. Today, and for the past several hundred years, the mantle has been worn by the Baptists. If we remain true, we may continue to wear it. If we do not, another group will be raised up, a people with a different name. But the name is not really important. If they stand for the same principles they will be the same people. "A rose by any other name would smell as sweet."

What's in a name? It depends on what we do, what we are, and what we stand for. Our ancestors made the name great. What the name means today is up to us!

BIBLIOGRAPHY

1. Verduin, Leonard, *The Reformers and Their Stepchildren*. Grand Rapids, Michigan: Baker Book House, 1980 P.B .

2. Armitage, Thomas, D.D., *History of the Baptists*. New York: Bryan, Taylor & Co., 1890. pp 1, 2

3. Good, Kenneth H., *God's Blueprint for a Church*. Des Plaines, Ill. : Regular Baptist Press, 1974. pp 119, 120

4. Martin, T. T., quoted by Mason, Roy, *The Church That Jesus Built*. Tampa, Fl. n.d., n.p. p 85

5. Good, ibid., p 120

6. Verduin, ibid., p 14

CHAPTER II
WHO SAID SO?

Baptists accept the Bible as their only sufficient authority for faith and practice. In general, this means the Scriptures of the Old and New Testaments. In particular, however, they look to the New Testament for most of their authority in their doctrine and practice. Believing this, we should cite some Scripture as our authority; and there are many. We shall consider only one in particular, that being the words of Paul to Timothy.

> All scripture is given by inspiration of God, and is profitable for doctrine, for reproof, for correction, for instruction in righteousness: That the man of God may be perfect, throughly furnished unto all good works.
>
> I charge thee therefore before God, and the Lord Jesus Christ, who shall judge the quick and the dead at his appearing and his kingdom; Preach the word; be instant in season, out of season; reprove, rebuke, exhort with all longsuffering and doctrine. For the time will come when they will not endure sound doctrine; but after their own lusts shall they heap to themselves teachers, having itching ears; and they shall turn away their ears from the truth, and shall be turned unto fables. But watch thou in all things, endure afflictions, do the work of an evangelist, make full proof of thy ministry (II Timothy 3:16-4:5).

How marvelously complete! Scripture is profitable and it is that upon which we are to base our doctrine: what we teach and therefore, what we believe. It is profitable and sufficient for reproof of those who have gone astray. It furnishes abundant correction for those who have erred. Further, it is the able instrument to be used for instruction in the way of righteousness. This is all accomplished by preaching the Word; and this includes reproving, rebuking, exhorting, and teaching.

Still using the Word, the preacher is to do the work of an evangelist and to make full proof of his ministry. Evidently he will be tested as to how well he has handled the Bible, the Word of God. The Bible is the substance and supply for the man of God. It is authoritative, and it is sufficient. Baptists believe this!

THE SACRED DESK

It is only reasonable, then, that Baptists would consider the preaching of the Bible to be the chief responsibility of the church. Worship, Christian education, and evangelism all revolve around this central function. It has been suggested that this is the reason, symbolically, that Baptists have one central pulpit and not one on either side of the platform, one for Bible reading and the other for preaching. One preacher, having observed the use of two pulpits, said he believed the reason for this practice was that "what was preached from the pulpit on one side of the platform could not be found in the Bible that was read at the pulpit on the other side of the platform." Historically, Baptists have demanded that their preachers preach the Word! The place that the Bible holds in Baptist life causes them to reject other things as authoritative, things that others accept. We shall consider some of them briefly.

WE'VE ALWAYS DONE IT THIS WAY

This is the cry that is raised many times when something new is suggested for the program of the church. It is also the reason that some churches believe and do what they do; it it tradition. The Jews in New Testament times were guilty of a form of this. Jesus said, "... Full well ye reject the commandment of God, that ye may keep your own tradition." (Mark 7:9). The tradition of which He spoke was the teaching of the scribes and Pharisees that set aside the teaching of the Law. Moses had commanded, "... Honour thy father and thy mother; ..." but tradition said that if a son had some wealth with which he might have helped his father and mother but he said to them, "It is Corban" (that is, a gift devoted to God) he would be free from his responsibility (Mark 7:10-11).

As it pertains to our discussion, tradition is defined in *The Shorter Oxford English Dictionary*, 1978 edition, as follows:

> In the Christian Church, any one, or the whole, of a body of teachings transmitted orally from generation to generation since early times: held by Roman Catholics to comprise *teaching derived from Christ and the apostles*, together with that subsequently communicated to the church by the Holy Spirit, and *to be of equal authority* with the Scripture. (Emphasis is mine.)

It should be noted that it is not always claimed by all who appeal to tradition that it is teaching derived from Christ and the apostles but simply that it is something that has been practiced for a long time. The claim is that it is time honored. However, many times the origin of the tradition has been lost in antiquity.

There is nothing wrong with tradition as such. For instance, Thanksgiving is a tradition, not in the above sense, but as being handed down from past generations. Perhaps there would be little wrong with observing teachings supposedly derived from Christ and the apostles if it were not for the fact that many of these traditions directly contradict their teachings that are recorded in the Bible. When this is true, tradition becomes heresy. Further, if these supposed teachings agree with Scripture, why would they be needed? Why not appeal directly to the Scriptures?

We could concede that tradition is all right, albeit unnecessary, if we observed tradition because it is valid; but when we say a thing is

A PEOPLE FOR HIS NAME

valid because it is a tradition, we are on dangerous ground. It is always safe to look only to the Scriptures, believing them to be sufficient.

COUNCILS, CREEDS, AND CONFESSIONS

Baptists also reject the decisions of church councils and the creeds that were formulated by them as being authoritative. Yet, it must be said that many of these councils and their creeds have been helpful in stating, in orderly fashion, the true teaching of Scripture on many important doctrines. Let us consider several of these councils.

The council of Nicaea, 325 A.D., was called by the emperor Constantine because of a theological debate that had been going on for some time between Arius and Athanasius. Arius thought that, since the heathen believed in many gods, for the Christians to believe that Jesus is God as well as the Father would mean that there are two Gods; therefore, the Christians would be going back into heathenism. He taught that Christ was something like God, but not God. He was a created being, first and highest of all, but still only a created being. He did not exist from eternity. He was not of the same essence with the Father. Sounds pretty much like present day Jehovah's Witnesses, doesn't it?

On the other hand, Athanasius held that Christ is very God. He said, "Jesus whom I know as my Redeemer, cannot be less than God."

More than three hundred bishops were present at the Nicene Council. Among them were some who bore the marks of the torture they had undergone for the sake of their faith. Their decision condemned the views of Arius, and they produced the first written creed of the church. However, the creed they adopted is not the one that is generally known as the Nicene Creed today, but a shorter one. Among other things the Nicene creed states, "Christ is very God of very God: begotten, not created; cosubstantial with the Father." There is nothing wrong with that, is there?

However, the Nicene Council had not addressed itself to all questions that were to arise. In the year 381 A.D., a second council convened in Constantinople. This council stood by the belief expressed in the Nicene Creed and, going further, declared its belief in the deity of the Holy Spirit. By doing this, the belief in the biblical doctrine of the Trinity was expressed.

More debate was to come as the church developed its doctrine in a more systematic way. Pelagianism is named after its founder, Pelagius, who taught against man's fall in Adam, original sin, man's total depravity, and predestination. Therefore, man is not born corrupt. Babies are innocent and only become bad as they grow up under the bad influence of others. Pretty good modern day liberalism, don't you think?

Pelagius was opposed by Augustine, so in 431 A.D., another council came together in Ephesus. Although Augustine died in 430 A.D., the Council of Ephesus condemned the teachings of Pelagius as heresy. This was a great step forward in expressing the biblical doctrines of sin and salvation. So far we would be hard put to find fault with the conclusions of the councils that we have mentioned.

Up to this time, however, the question of the humanity of Jesus had not been addressed. In the Bible, Jesus is portrayed as being human as well as divine, man as well as God. This matter also brought forth much difference of opinion.

In 451 A.D., a council was held in Chalcedon near Nicaea. In the creed which they produced, they reaffirmed their belief in the deity of Jesus and went still further to declare their belief in His humanity and that He had two natures, human and divine; but He was just one person.[1]

Baptists would not reject these truths we have noticed, truths that were expressed by these councils and their creeds. In fact, many Baptists quote from them in expressing their own beliefs. However, they do not appeal to them as authority for their beliefs. To them, councils and creeds are correct only as they reflect the teachings of the Word of God. They do not necessarily see anything wrong with giving, in written form, a statement of their belief concerning the teaching of Scrip-

A PEOPLE FOR HIS NAME

ture. To Baptists, creeds are just that and no more.

Baptists have, in fact, produced some rather elaborate creeds of their own. They call them confessions of faith. Most notable among them are the *London Confession* which was patterned after the *Westminster Confession*, and its American form, the *Philadelphia Confession*. Both of these were quite detailed statements of what these Baptists believed. The *New Hampshire Confession* was produced at a later date and is the one that is accepted by many Baptists in the United States, in the North and in the South. It is much less detailed than the two mentioned above.

In spite of these confessions, Baptists seem at times, to have had an aversion to setting down what they believed in written form. When the Southern Baptist Convention came into being in 1845 they did not make a statement of faith. They said, "We have constructed for our basis no new creed, acting in this matter upon a Baptist aversion for all creeds except the Bible."[2]

So, whether they had creeds or not, they have consistently rejected councils, creeds, or confessions as being authoritative in matters of faith and practice. To them, it is all right to accept creeds as expressions of what they believe but not as authority for what they believe. That is found only in the Bible.

HIERARCHAL UTTERANCES

Some churches look to a hierarchy, a body of persons ranked in order or classes one above another, as their final authority in matters of faith and practice. When those of the higher order speak, this becomes their doctrine. This is notably true in the Roman Catholic Church. To Catholics, the Pope is the highest order. He is believed to be infallible when he speaks, ex cathedra, in matters of the Church. Although they believe him to be divinely protected, so that he could make a decision alone, greater external solemnity is given to the Church's decrees when all her bishops, jointly with the Pope, make the decision.

However it is done, the utterance is from those higher up and is official. It might be a mixture of something a past council has said, tradition, something extra-biblical that they claim has been handed down from Jesus and the apostles or the church fathers and that contradicts the Bible or is absent from the teachings of Scripture; but if the Church has spoken, that is the way it is. Again, let it be said that Baptists reject this. No human being can be the authority for what another is to believe. This must come from Scripture.

SOLA SCRIPTURA

Strangely, however, it seems that some agree with the Baptists on this matter; at least that is what they claim. Sola Scriptura, only Scripture or Scripture alone, was Luther's watchword and pretty much became the watchword of the Reformation. After all, it was to the Scriptures that Luther appealed for his doctrine of *Justification by Faith*. A little later we will see just how closely Luther and the Reformers adhered to this.

The Catholic Church, on the other hand, does not even claim to look only to the Bible. For them, the Bible does not contain all that God has revealed. Further revelation is found in the writings of the early church fathers, the decrees of church councils, the decisions of the Pope, etc. That takes in just about everything and leaves room for teaching just about anything. These things constitute the tradition that we talked about earlier; and this gave rise to all kinds of strange doctrine, things that are foreign to the teachings of Scripture.

FROM THE ROOT TO THE FRUIT

Since this system that we have just considered leaves room for teaching just about anything, we need to pause and notice some of the teachings and practices that resulted from it. It should be noticed that such a system as this results in one never being able to be certain of all that Catholics believe. If they feel the need for additional teaching on any subject they have only to appeal to one of their sources and ... voila! Sort of like making up the rules as you play the game.

On the other hand, we shall soon discover that the Reformers did not stick too closely to the Scriptures in some matters, and this caused many problems between them and the predecessors of the Baptists.

To deal with all of the doctrines and practices of the Catholic Church that resulted from their many sources of revelation would be impossible in the scope of this chapter. We shall discuss enough of them to show that they certainly were not revealed in the Bible. Many of them are those that have been most relevant to the subject of Baptist distinctives. As we have seen, Baptists and Catholics are at the extreme opposite ends of the field as to the source of their doctrine. Because of this there were definite doctrinal differences that resulted in the severe persecution of those who held many of our distinctives.

Consider first some Catholic teachings concerning Mary, the mother of Jesus. They are her *Immaculate Conception*, her *Perpetual Virginity*, and her *Bodily Assumption*.

The *Immaculate Conception* means that Mary was conceived in such a way as to preserve her from original sin, i.e., that which all human beings partake of by natural generation. In this way Jesus could be protected from original sin since she had none to pass on to Him. The Bible is silent concerning this. However, since our fallen, sinful nature comes from our father, Adam, and not from our mother, Eve, it seems that this nature would be passed from father to child and would not be received from the mother. If this is true, the virgin birth of Jesus would have protected Him from any original sin, since He received nothing from a human father. It looks as if the problem might have been solved before the "powers that be" got around to it.

Mary's *Perpetual Virginity* means that, not only was Mary a virgin at the time Jesus was conceived and when He was born, she remained a virgin for the remainder of her life. The only part of this that can be substantiated from Scripture is that she was a virgin at the time of the conception and birth of Jesus and that Joseph "... knew her not till she had brought forth her firstborn son: . . ." (Matthew 1:25). This at least implies that he did "know" her after Jesus was born. Further, the New Testament speaks several times of the brethren of Jesus (Matthew 12:46, John 2:12, etc.). This seems to be an obvious contradiction of the notion that she remained a virgin for the remainder of her life.

But why would it matter whether Mary remained a virgin for the rest of her life or not. That she was a virgin at the time of the conception of Jesus and at His birth is important, among other reasons, because it fulfills Old Testament prophecy. However, there is no biblical reason that she should remain a perpetual virgin.

In the view of the Catholic Church this is a different matter. Influenced as it is by Augustinian Platonism it sees sex, even in the bonds of marriage, as something less than pure. While Augustine was not a total Platonist, he did display a notorious contempt for the material. He is said to have described marriage as "the reputable enjoyment of voluptuousness." That the Roman Catholic Church follows this vein of thought is seen in a statement of Pope John Paul II as reported in *Time Magazine*. According to this source, he said that if a man looked lustfully even ". . . at the woman who is his wife, he could commit adultery 'in his heart' " (*Time*, October 27, 1980, p. 106).[3]

For the Catholic, sexual pleasure within marriage is to be sought only for the propagation of the race. Otherwise, man acts contrary to the will of God. Hence, the stand against birth control. Following this line of thinking, they would have to believe that there is something wrong with the normal function of marriage between a man and his wife. This explains the necessity, in the Catholic's way of thinking, for the doctrine of the *Perpetual Virginity of Mary*.

But the Word of God, the Bible says, "Marriage is honourable in all, and the bed undefiled: . . ." (Hebrews 13:4). Further sex in marriage is prescribed by the Apostle Paul as a means of control of the fires of sexual passion (I Corinthians 7:1-9).

Following the teaching of Augustine, one of the church fathers, as a source of revelation upon which to build the dogma of the Church certainly made shipwreck on this one.

The doctrine of Mary's *Bodily Assumption* is that, when she died, her body was received into heaven without seeing corruption. But, hold the press! I remember reading in the newspaper some thirty years ago that the "Holy Father" was saying that Mary went to heaven without dying. Later, as I recall, this teaching was retracted because there was so much objection to it. Well, I figured I should check this out, so I called the local Catholic priest. When I told him what I thought I remembered reading he, unabashedly, said that it was true; not only was she assumed into heaven, but she went without dying. He did say that there were not too many references to this event in the Bible. I asked how many, and he said he did not know of any. Neither do I!!! I then asked him how long this had been a teaching of the Church, and he said that it had been a tradition for quite some time.

He then explained that this was possible because of her immaculate conception. Since there was no sin, she did not die. You will search the Scriptures in vain for this one.

To these teachings, add that Mary is the mother of God. Now it is true that Mary was the mother of Jesus. It is also true that Jesus is God. However, the *logos*, the Word, was in existence as God from eternity. Mary bore the earthly body of Jesus at a point in time. Only in this sense is Mary the mother of our Lord; she is not the mother of the eternal God. Neither is she "queen of heaven." In the Old Testament book of Jeremiah this designation is used several times in connection with pagan worship (Jeremiah 44:17-25).

Catholics are taught to pray to Mary in order to get her to intercede with God for them. The reasoning is that no one would have more compassion on the petitioner than a woman and that no one would have more influence with the Son than His mother. Yet Jesus is portrayed in Scripture as being filled with compassion. He is also presented as the "... one mediator between God and men, ..." (I Timothy 2:5).

We shall now turn our attention to some other teachings of the Catholic Church, the doctrine of *Purgatory* and the doctrine of *Tran-*

substantiation. Both of these doctrines result from extra-biblical sources and they strike directly at the heart of the biblical teaching of the completeness of the work of Jesus on the cross.

Purgatory is a place where souls go after death and before they go on to heaven. So says the Catholic Church. The reason is that only the very good can expect to go to heaven immediately after death and only the very bad deserve hell. There must be some place for those in between to go, and that place is purgatory. It is the place to which those who die with small sins unatoned for must go to be punished for a time.

Catholics even have a Scripture verse for this one, Matthew 5:26. But read the context and you will never get purgatory out of it without the help of a priest. The verse obviously refers to a debtors' prison here on earth, not to purgatory after death.

It can readily be seen that this doctrine teaches that the blood of Jesus is not able to atone for all of our sins. It also teaches that there is something we must do in order to be among those who can go directly to heaven, and that those who go to purgatory have failed to do sufficient penance for their sins. If only they had done more! So sins must be atoned for on earth by doing more. If they are not, they must be atoned for after death by someone doing more; either the one in purgatory must suffer more, or more prayers must be said, or someone must pay the priest to say masses to obtain an uncertain release from purgatory. This is salvation by works and it makes a mockery of the doctrine of *Justification by Grace Through Faith* since ". . . if it be of works, then it is no more grace: . . ." (Romans 11:6). It makes salvation a deserved commodity. But grace is the unmerited favor of God.

In addition, this doctrine contradicts the writings of the apostle Paul in II Corinthians 5:1-8, where he leaves the idea that a Christian who is absent from the body is immediately present with the Lord. See also Philippians 1:23 where Paul expresses a desire to ". . . depart, and to be with Christ; . . . ." This seems to be a misguided aspiration if he has to lay over in purgatory for an indeterminate period of time. Clearly, this doctrine is the result of looking to non-biblical sources as the authority in faith and practice.[a]

We shall now consider the doctrine of *Transubstantiation*, which caused no little persecution at the hands of those who held it. It has to do with the Lord's Supper, communion; and it was incorporated into the Catholic's *"Sacrifice of the Mass."* The teaching is that when the priests say the sacramental words, the bread and wine of the supper actually turn into the body and blood of Jesus, notwithstanding the fact that there is no outward change in these elements. Having accomplished this miracle, they can sacrifice Jesus again and again and again, thus making a continual sacrifice. No wonder Martin Luther broke into a cold sweat the first time he tried this one.

Obviously, Catholics take the words, "... this is my body" and "... this is my blood ..." (Matthew 26:26, 28) literally. However, it can

---

[a]Shedd, William, G. T., *A History of Christian Doctrine*, New York, New York: Charles Scribner's Sons, 1884. Vol. II of 2 Vols. pp 255, 410, 411

According to Shedd, the doctrine of purgatory was intimately connected with that of an intermediate state and was developed along with it. A belief in the intermediate state was held by several of the early fathers. The doctrine of purification of believers who had become partially sanctified in this life shows itself as early as the 4th century. Augustine supposes that the teachings of Paul in I Cor. 3:11-15 imply that the remainder of corruption in the renewed soul may be purged away in the period between death and the final judgment. The idea of purifying fire is distinctly presented by Gregory Nazianzen, but the Papal doctrine in its full form does not appear until the time of Gregory the Great (604 A.D.). He gave it as an article of faith, and was the first writer who clearly propounded the idea of a deliverance from purgatory by intercessory prayer and masses for the dead.

Earlier in his book, Shedd wrote, "Augustine sometimes confuses Justification with Sanctification." Justification is an instantaneous act of God whereby He declares the believing sinner to be just. While Sanctification is also instantaneous in one sense, in another it is progressive and will only be complete when we "...see him as he is" (John 3:2). Confusing these two doctrines could have led Augustine to his erroneous conclusion that further purification was needed after death.

When a person builds upon his own error or the error of another, error is compounded as in the case of the full grown doctrine of purgatory.

readily be seen that Jesus was speaking symbolically since He was present in His flesh when He presented the bread and the cup to the disciples. Jesus spoke symbolically when He said, "I am the door . . ." (John 10:9). Certainly, these words are not to be taken literally. Paul also uses symbolic language. He wrote, "For as often as ye eat this bread, and drink this cup, . . ." (I Corinthians 11:26). But he did not mean that we literally drink the cup. We drink what is in it and we all understand that when we read it. Even so, the bread is a symbol of His body and the cup, of his blood. We are to eat the bread and drink the wine, that and nothing more. As we do this, we can be certain that it is bread we are eating and wine we are drinking, not the body and blood of Jesus.[4]

The doctrine of Transubstantiation is a serious departure from the teaching of Scripture for several reasons. First, it denies the efficacy of the one sacrifice that Jesus made on the cross. Jesus ". . . offered one sacrifice for sins for ever, . . ." (Hebrews 10:12). He will never offer another one, nor does one need to be made. Sinners are saved on the basis of that one sacrifice and not one that is offered over and over again.

Further, to Catholics, this is a necessary means of grace, and a priest is necessary since only priests are empowered to turn the bread and wine into the flesh and blood of Jesus. Thus, he becomes a sacrificing priest, and this gives a great solemnity to the term "excommunication." One who has been excommunicated would be excluded from participating in a mass that could aid in salvation, bring good fortune in a business venture, shorten the time he spends in purgatory, etc. Now you can see why excommunication is feared so much and what power it gives the priest over the people since to be without access to a priest is to be without access to this means of grace. You can also see why Baptists have stood vehemently against this doctrine.

UNREFORMED REFORMERS

When the Reformation began there seemed to be a general turning of the Reformers to a position that favored the Bible as the only sufficient source of revelation and authority for faith and practice. Remember Luther's watchword, "Sola Scriptura." Further evidence is found in his declaration at the "Diet of Worms." He said, "... My conscience is bound to the Word of God.... Here I stand. God help me. I cannot do otherwise "

But how did he stand in actual practice? Was he willing to let the Scriptures be authoritative and look only to them as the sole basis for his doctrine? Apparently not! Verduin writes,

> Luther was likewise embarrassed with "christening." But he was too well aware of the radicalness of a clean break.... Wrote he: "There is not sufficient evidence from Scripture that one might justify the introduction of infant baptism at the time of the early Christians after the apostolic period.... But so much is evident, that no one may venture with a good conscience to reject or abandon infant baptism, *which has for so long a time been practiced.*"[5] (Emphasis is mine.)

This sounds pretty much like an appeal to tradition in order to circumvent what he felt was the real teaching of Scripture. Verduin reports further that the Reformer Oecolampadius said, "I know only too well that you keep calling 'Scripture, Scripture!' as you clamor for clear words to prove our point.... But if Scripture taught us all things then there would be no need for the anointing to teach us all things."[6]

Of course, the anointing does teach us all things (I John 2:27); but it does it in conjunction with the word of God. It teaches us nothing apart from the Word. The belief that this Reformer held was evidently that the anointing taught things that the Word does not and that would leave him an unlimited source of revelation on which to build his doctrine of whatever. The late Dr. Charles H. Stevens, founder of Piedmont Bible College and for many years its president, used to say that it was all right to put your antenna up in order to receive special revelations as long as that antenna was firmly grounded in God's Word.

At first Ulrich Zwingli, the Swiss Reformer, turned to and accepted the "Bible only" principle, according to many historians. He admitted that he was inclined to reject infant baptism, which would have been logical if he looked only to the Scriptures for authority for his belief. But Zwingli was in bondage to the idea of a State-Church. He felt that, for the Reformation to succeed, the power of the civil government was necessary. For the State-Church union to succeed, infant baptism was a necessity. So he turned from the Bible as authority and accepted that which was expedient. As a result Zwingli became a persecutor of those who rejected infant baptism and who baptized only those who professed salvation. We shall see more about this in a later chapter.

We will go no further at this time in showing that the Reformers did not always look only to the Scriptures as their authority. This practice will be seen to have affected their relationship with our ancestors. What we need to consider now is that if this could happen to the Reformers, it could also happen to those of us today who claim to look only to Scripture.

BLOCKING BAPTIST BLUNDERS

If, in any way, we circumvent the plain teaching of Scripture we will inevitably turn to some other source as our authority. To prevent this, let us consider several ways that are frequently practiced today to avoid the plain teaching of the Bible.

HUMAN REASON: The Word of God has been summoned to appear before the bar of reason. This is seen in the attempt of the Jehovah's Witnesses to dismiss the doctrine of a burning hell. They say, among other things, that it is unreasonable. Of course, this is the result of human reasoning, that plus plain unbelief. They have placed Scripture in the crucible of human reason and it failed their test. So they reject the teaching of Scripture and their reason becomes their final

A PEOPLE FOR HIS NAME

authority.[a]

DATING SCRIPTURE: This is done when a person explains that certain scriptural standards were right when they were written but that times have changed. This would mean that the standards of right and wrong were arrived at by examining the existing environment or by looking at certain cultures to see what standards were best for them. When cultures changed, so did the standards. But cultures do change, and that means that we could have no absolute standards of right and wrong. What would be right in one culture would be wrong in another. This is akin to situation ethics, and what is best in a given situation becomes the final authority. Since the individual must make a judgment based upon the circumstances, he is supreme. Exit God's Word!

POLL TAKING: A common cry among teenagers and adults alike who want to indulge in some worldly activity is "everybody is doing it." This is supposed to make anything all right regardless of what the Bible says. But if everyone is doing something that is sin, this makes a common desire and a willingness to disobey God's will the final authority. But remember, as long as you are not doing this thing, the claim that everybody is doing it is a lie.

INTERPRETING THE WORD: Of course, this is necessary.

---

[a] Throckmorton, Burton Jr., "NCC's Bisexual Lectionary Brings More Problems," *Christianity Today*, December 16, 1983

"The Scripture is the church's book. It was written by the church (and) for the church," Throckmorton said. "There's no reason...that I can see why the church can't add to its Scripture--delete from its Scripture. I think the church can do with its Scripture what it wants to (do) with its Scripture."

This is an example of men blatantly sitting in judgment of the Word of God. They become the final authority and they can make Scripture say what they want it to say and not say that which is displeasing to them.

Throckmorton is a member of the committee that produced the bisexual version of the Bible. He is professor of New Testament at the Bangor (Maine) Theological Seminary, and a minister in the Presbyterian Church (U.S.A.).

However, there is a right way and wrong way to do it. One method is to decide what you want to believe and then interpret the Bible to fit. The other way is to study the Scriptures in order to find what you ought to believe. The first method makes your belief the authority. Human reason and rationalization are often used to interpret God's Word in a way that suits us.

IGNORING THE WORD: If a person ignores enough for long enough he is ignorant. Being ignorant of the Bible prevents us from being doers of the Word. But to know the message of the Bible and then ignore it is worse. This is sin. "Therefore to him that knoweth to do good, and doeth it not, to him it is sin" (James 4:17). This certainly keeps the Bible from being the only sufficient authority in matters of faith and practice.

May we learn from the mistakes of others so that we may continue to be a people who look only to the Bible as our authority, believing that it is all we need.

BIBLIOGRAPHY

1. Kuiper, B. K., *The Church in History*. Grand Rapids, Michigan: Wm. B. Eerdmans Publishing Co., 1951 pp 56-58 ; 73-76. Summary

2. Barnes, W. W., *The Southern Baptist Convention*, 1845-1953. Nashville, Tennessee: Broadman Press, 1954. p. 118

3. Pinell, E. A., "Augustine's Neo-Platonism," *Christian Newsletter*, May 1981. Summary

4. Boettner, Loraine, *Roman Catholicism*. I understand this work is now published by Baker Book House. See it for a more complete discussion of the Mass and Transubstantiation.

5. Verduin, Leonard, *The Reformers and Their Stepchildren*. Grand Rapids, Michigan: Baker Book House, 1964. pp 203-204

6. Ibid., p 204

CHAPTER III
FAMILY AFFAIR

Obviously, no one would believe that anyone was a member of a certain family, or had a right to be, unless that person had been born into that family or had been properly and legally adopted. Just as obvious is the teaching of the New Testament concerning church membership. If we approach the study of the New Testament without preconceived ideas or theological assumptions and look to it alone as our authority, we will come to the conclusion that a New Testament church consists only of those who have been born again, i.e., those who are regenerate. Therefore, Baptists believe in a regenerate church membership. Being born again is a family affair.

Yet, it was not very late in the history of the church when unregenerate folks were found in it. Later, a belief developed among some Christians that the unsaved ought to be included in its membership.

Talk about a "mixt multitude!" If you think the one back in Moses' time (Numbers 11) caused problems just wait until we consider all the results and ramifications of this one.

The real beginning of this problem can be traced to the emperor Constantine's dubious conversion to Christianity. Since this will affect the church greatly, let's look at it carefully. In 306 A.D., Constantine had been proclaimed emperor by the army in Britain. He was now ruler over Britain, Gaul (which is now France), and Spain. However, Maxentius ruled over Italy and North Africa; and he wanted to rule over all of the western part of the Roman Empire. Needless to say, a great deal of hostility existed between these two men. Before Maxentius could make preparation for war, Constantine got the jump on him and marched into Italy with an army of forty thousand men. They met at the Milvian Bridge which crossed the Tiber River about ten miles from

Rome. Here a problem became apparent to Constantine; the army of Maxentius had more than one hundred thousand men and contained crack troops known as the Praetorian Guards.

Constantine found himself in a very precarious position. He must have realized the need of supernatural help, and being a worshiper of Mithra, the Persian sun-god, evidently sought help from him. However, on the afternoon of the day before the battle, Constantine saw, above the sun, a cross with the words *hoc signo vinces*, which means "in this sign, conquer." He understood this to mean that if he would embrace Christianity, he would be victorious. The day of the battle was October 28; the year was 312 A.D. The battle was furiously fought; and although the troops of Maxentius fought well, Constantine was victorious. Maxentius was drowned as he attempted to escape over the Milvian Bridge. Constantine was now ruler of the entire western part of the Roman Empire, and he felt that he had been victorious because he received help from the Christians' God. He embraced Christianity; and his edict of Milan, 313 A.D., placed Christianity on an equal basis with the other religions of the Empire. Sitting on the throne, there was now a man who claimed to be a Christian. Persecution of Christians ceased, and it was no longer a shame to be a Christian. Christianity became popular.[1] As a result, many heathen people joined the church, people who knew nothing of the New Birth. At best they had been christianized. Certainly, they were not regenerate. Therefore, they knew nothing of the indwelling Holy Spirit to teach them and lead them into all truth.

It was only natural that a church composed partly of unregenerate people would soon be affected by their thinking, thinking that was of the world because they were of the world. Since they were unsaved, they would think it proper that others like themselves should be members. What began in practice soon became church dogma. A concept was born that was foreign to early Christians; namely, that a church consists of all in a given locality, saved and unsaved alike. Early Christians had held that the church was to consist only of those who had exercised personal faith in Jesus and had received Him as their Lord and Saviour.

Results of this were to be serious and far reaching, affecting the church throughout much of its history. It is almost impossible to discuss the Baptists' belief in a regenerate church membership and this opposite belief without getting into a discussion of the State-Church issue since both issues are so closely related. However, since we want to discuss the State-Church controversy in detail in a later chapter, we will try to confine our discussion to the make-up of a biblical church.

BIBLE BASES FOR A REGENERATE CHURCH MEMBERSHIP

As we consider why Baptists believe as they do concerning this important subject, it is important that we caution everyone, especially Baptists, against accepting any belief just because Baptists hold it. The reason for any belief must be that it is biblical. We shall soon see that those who have held to the idea of a church consisting of all in a given locality must look to extrabiblical sources, as must those who believe that infants are proper subjects for membership. But what about Baptists? Why do they believe as they do? Do they have biblical proof for their belief in a regenerate church membership?

There is definite evidence that the early church believed it was to be responsible for the purity of its membership. That is, its members were to see that only those who were genuinely saved were allowed to be baptized. It seems to be agreed upon by most that baptism, in one form or another, is a prerequisite to church membership. Accordingly, we find evidence that the church could refuse baptism and, therefore, church membership to one who had not met certain criteria. What were these criteria?

The first baptismal service of the church is recorded in the second chapter of the book of Acts. There we read, "Then they that gladly received his word were baptized: and the same day there were added

A PEOPLE FOR HIS NAME

unto them about three thousand souls" (Acts 2:41). Conversely, had they not "gladly received his word" they would not have been admitted to the ordinance of baptism, nor would they have been added to the church. The reason is simple. Receiving his word, i.e., that which Peter had preached, the gospel, was the same as believing unto salvation. Had they not done so they would not have been regenerate and therefore, not qualified for membership in the church. This, alone, is enough on which to base the doctrine of a regenerate church membership. But there is more. During Philip's citywide campaign in Samaria those who "... believed Philip preaching the things concerning the kingdom of God, and the name of Jesus Christ, ... were baptized, ..." (Acts 8:12). It is not so stated, but they evidently became members of the church. However, the fact that they believed as they did gives evidence that they were regenerate. Had they not been, they would not have been admitted to the ordinance of baptism and would not have been considered to be qualified for church membership.

It might be argued by some that they did not receive the Holy Spirit until the apostles from Jerusalem laid their hands on them. However, remember that this is the first complete record of the gospel being preached outside of Jerusalem. The normal course of the age had not been reached. This would come about later as Peter preached the gospel in the house of Cornelius.

At that time, after Peter had preached the death and resurrection of Jesus, he said, "To him give all the prophets witness, that through his name whosoever believeth in him shall receive remission of sins" (Acts 10:43). While Peter was still speaking, "... the Holy Ghost fell on all them which heard the word" (Acts 10:44). A careful study of the context shows that those who heard did not just hear audibly. They heard with approval; they believed what Peter said and, believing, they were saved. Therefore, when Peter asked, "Can any man forbid water, that these should not be baptized, which have received the Holy Ghost as well as we?" (Acts 10:47), none objected. The reason? They had seen evidence that they believed and were regenerate. They were qualified for church membership!

That the Holy Ghost fell on those to whom Peter was preaching and who "heard the word" was evidence that they believed what he was preaching and that they were regenerate. Had this not been evident to Peter and to the brethren who were with him, they would have forbidden them the water of baptism. They would not have been deemed to be qualified for membership in the church.

In Romans, instructions are given to receive one who is ". . . weak in the faith . . ." (Romans 14:1). But there must be faith of some sort and that would imply regeneration. Even the beloved apostle Paul had a hard time joining the local church at Jerusalem. The reason was that the disciples, who were members, ". . . were all afraid of him, and believed not that he was a disciple" (Acts 9:26). If they had believed that he was a disciple, they would not have been afraid of him and he would have been readily accepted. It was because they did not believe that he believed that they did not think him a fit candidate for church membership.

Although II Corinthians 6 goes beyond the scope of church membership, it certainly teaches that there is no basis for regenerate and unregenerate people to be members of the same church. Paul gave the following instructions and logic:

> Be ye not unequally yoked together with unbelievers: for what fellowship hath righteousness with unrighteousness? and what communion hath light with darkness? And what concord hath Christ with Belial? or what part hath he that believeth with an infidel? And what agreement hath the temple of God with idols? for ye are the temple of the living God; as God hath said, I will dwell in them, and walk in them; and I will be their God, and they shall be my people (II Corinthians 6:14-16).

The answer to each of these questions is a resounding "none." Believers and unbelievers have no common ground for unity, especially in the church. Accordingly, in the verses that follow, instructions are given to "... come out from among them, and be ye separate, ..." (II Corinthians 6:17).

There is also ample evidence in Scripture that, not only did God intend for His church to be composed of regenerate people, He also intended that they should live as if they were regenerate. Believers who constituted the church were responsible to watch over fellow believers in this matter and to exercise discipline when necessary. The Corinthian Church is a classical example of this. In response to the gross sin in their midst, the apostle Paul said emphatically, "Purge out therefore the old leaven, that ye may be a new lump, as ye are unleavened..." (I Corinthians 5:7). Leaven, in this context, is evil. Continuing, Paul speaks more plainly concerning what they were to do with one among them who was guilty of sin. He wrote that they should "... deliver such an one unto Satan for the destruction of the flesh, that the spirit may be saved in the day of the Lord Jesus" (I Corinthians 5:5). Further, he said, "... Therefore put away from among yourselves that wicked person" (I Corinthians 5:13). There can be no doubt, God desires a pure church.

Certainly, enough evidence has been presented from the Bible to show that only one who is regenerate is to be a member of the church. It is definitely true that God adds only this kind of person and it is just as true that, as much as possible, believers should admit only those who believe. Therefore, Baptists have historically believed that only those who profess to have believed, savingly, in Jesus and who give evidence of having been regenerated, born again, are proper subjects for membership in a New Testament church. In view of all the biblical evidence to the contrary, we are made to wonder why anyone would believe that a New Testament church should be composed of saved and unsaved alike. Let's look now at some things that have resulted in unsaved church members.

CONSTANTINE

As we have seen, the real beginning of this practice of accepting unregenerate members into the church can be traced to the Constantine caper. Several things about him and the condition of his empire help to explain why his reign resulted in this practice.

First, Constantine's conversion is seen by a number of historians as doubtful, at best. While some are not willing to say he was never really converted, many express doubts. Although it is difficult to be sure whether his conversion to Christianity was genuine or not, there are several reasons for doubting it. He evidently believed in Baptismal Regeneration and that salvation could be lost, since he delayed his own baptism until a time just before his death. He became Pontifex Maximus, or chief priest, of the Christian church; but he retained his position of Pontifex Maximus of the pagan state religion. Further, his practice of executing young men who could have laid claim to his throne is not exactly in keeping with the morality of a true Christian. Therefore, if he was not a genuine Christian, he would not have had spiritual understanding of a church composed only of the regenerate. This would certainly have set the stage for an influx of the unregenerate.

Second, it appears that his motives in what he did might have been more political than Christian. While some are not willing to concede that his actions were simply a matter of political expediency, they still feel that his motives are open to question. The empire over which Constantine ruled was in trouble. It was coming apart and was in need of something to stabilize it. Cairns is of the opinion that

> . . . it is likely that Constantine's favoritism to the Church was a matter of expediency. The Church might serve as a new center of unity and save classical culture and the Empire.[2]

Verduin believes

> ... the problem to which Constantine sought a solution was political rather than religious .... The empire he had inherited was coming apart at the seams .... How could he conquer this problem? Then came the much celebrated "vision," a cross in the clouds, and the words "in hoc signo vinces" (in this sign conquer). There he had it! Make the religion of Jesus the religion of the empire and then look to it to achieve the consensus that he, sacralist that he was, and remained, felt he had to have.[3]

If this assumption is correct and if his plan was to have a reasonable chance of success, the emperor would have to have as many as possible committed to Christianity in one way or another. This being the case, it would not matter too much to him whether they were saved or unsaved, regenerate or unregenerate. This would be a definite detriment to any safeguard that would keep the church pure.

Third, before Constantine accepted Christianity, he had been a worshiper of Mithra, the Persian sun-god, as his father before him had been. After his conversion, Constantine outlawed Sunday work, thus setting Sunday apart as a day of rest and worship. But to him, influenced as he was as a worshiper of the sun-god, Sunday was the "Day of the Sun."[a] So even if he had some Christian motivation in outlawing Sunday work, there is a distinct possibility that there is a motivation that was left over from Mithra worship. The point is this: Constantine was still influenced by his first religion, a religion that had no parallel to Christian regeneration. Therefore, he would have little, if any, understanding of the necessity of the new birth for one who was to become a candidate for baptism and church membership.

---

[a]Notice, this was not the origin of Sunday worship. Christians do not worship on Sunday because Constantine set the day aside. If he had a Christian motive, he set the day aside because Christians already worshipped on that day. Sunday was the day of Christian worship since earliest New Testament times. See Acts 20:6-7 as an example.

Remember, Constantine was Pontifex Maximus of the church; and what affected him would doubtless have a profound effect on the doctrine and practice of the church. Add to this the fact that he was very generous in the monetary subsidization of the church, and you can see what great influence he wielded over the clergy. After all, the one who pays the fiddler calls the tune.

STATE-CHURCH, COERCION, AND INFANT BAPTISM

From what we have just discussed, we can see something of the beginning of the belief and practice of allowing unregenerate people to become members of the church. However, we must not think that this was developed in one fell swoop, or apart from other results. Its full development was over a period of many years and its ramifications were many. Things got worse. In the course of time a practice developed of coercing people to be baptized and become members on pain of confiscation of property, banishment, torture, and even death by the most horrendous means. This was bound to result in many unregenerate people coming into the church, and that is exactly what happened.

Coercion was a part of the result of the State-Church concept that we mentioned earlier and, as we have stated, the doctrine and practice of infant baptism were looked upon by a number of the Reformers, and others, as absolutely necessary if the State-Church idea was to succeed.

At this point, we will only discuss infant baptism to show that baptized infants do become members of the church and that this would result in unregenerate members. Adams writes,

> ... It is an undeniable fact, that all Pedobaptist churches [infant baptizers] have contended that infants are proper subjects for membership in the church, and therefore should be baptized. There are two opinions, however, as to the grounds of infant bap-

tism. Some contend that the infants of professed believers should be baptized because they are already members of the church, by their natural birth, while others contend that they should be baptized in order to make them members. All Pedobaptists, however, agree, that infants are proper subjects for church membership, and by baptism they receive such to their membership....[4]

Further, Adams quotes from the Westminster Confession of Faith, the Larger Catechism, and the Discipline of the Presbyterian Church in the United States as follows:

... The Presbyterian Confession of Faith says: "The visible church consists of all those throughout the world that profess the true religion, together with their children." We are told again, that "Baptism is a sacrament," "whereby the parties baptized are solemnly admitted into the visible church." "All baptized persons are members of the church, are under its care, and subject to its government and discipline, and *when they have arrived at years of discretion*, they are bound to perform all the duties of church members" (emphasis is his).[5]

One other quotation should suffice to show that infants are considered proper subjects for baptism and church membership. In view of the two previous quotations, the following statement by Louis Berkhof implies that he believes that infants should become members of the church. Notice the following excerpt:

... Baptism is intended for believers and their seed. Only rational beings, ... are proper subjects of baptism. There are two classes to whom baptism is applied, namely, adults and infants.[6]

And that, of course, takes in just about everybody!

Now, no one would claim that these little babies would cause a great deal of trouble in the church as far as its doctrine, policy, or practice is concerned. But remember, "When they have arrived at years of discretion, they are bound to perform all the duties of church members." If, at that time, they still have not been born again there is cause for serious concern. According to Adams, et al, there seems to be a reluctance to cut off from membership those who have become members of the church in infancy, even though there is a lack of evidence of regeneration in their lives and, at times, definite evidence to the contrary.

How can Baptists be so dogmatic in their stand concerning the matter of babies becoming members of the church, a stand with which so many differ greatly? The reason is that, according to Scripture, salvation is by grace through faith. Faith is belief, and infants cannot believe savingly. There is nothing in Scripture about parents believing for their children. If this were necessary, important, or even possible, certainly there would be something about it somewhere in the Bible. Therefore, even infants who have been baptized are unregenerate and are not qualified for membership in a New Testament church. However, they are safe, as we shall see later.

Notice, the thrust of this section is not concerned with the rightness or wrongness of infant baptism as such. What has been written here is simply meant to show its relationship to the views of those who do not believe that the church should consist only of those who are regenerated and to show that infant baptism does result in some unregenerated people in the membership of churches.

UNDEFINED DISPENSATIONAL DIFFERENCE

Going further, a lack of understanding of the dispensational difference between the Old Testament and the New Testament is greatly responsible for the unregenerate being considered as properly belonging in the church. For those who hold Covenant Theology, the New Testament church is simply a continuation of Old Testament Israel. Every person in the Old Testament society was considered to be in the same position, religiously, as was every other person. Carry this over into New Testament theology, and the logical conclusion would be that every person should be in the New Testament society, the church. The result of such thinking would, of course, be unsaved church members.

UNEXAMINED PROFESSIONS

A further reason that unsaved folks are found in the membership of many churches is that some obviously do not take proper care to ascertain that professions of faith are genuine. In fairness to those of the reformed faith, I will quote their stand, which requires a profession on the part of adults before they are admitted to membership. Berkhof writes,

> ... In the case of adults baptism must be preceded by a profession of faith, Acts 8:37; ... Mark 16:16; Acts 2:41; 16:31-33. Therefore the Church insists on such a profession before baptizing adults....[7]

However, Berkhof disclaims any real responsibility on the part of the church to ascertain the genuineness of such a profession. He continues,

> ... And when such a profession is made, this is accepted by the Church at its face value, unless there are phenomena which cause her to doubt its veracity. It does not belong to her province to pry into the secrets of the heart and thus pass on the genuineness of such a profession ... The method of prying into the inner condition of the heart, in order to determine the genuineness of one's profession, is Labadistic and not in harmony with the practice of the Reformed Churches....[8]

Such a stand is consistent with the view that the unregenerate are proper subjects for church membership.

However, Scripture is replete with statements that indicate that the condition of the heart can be known by examining a person's outward action. Consider the following: "For as he thinketh in his heart, so is he: ..." (Proverbs 23:7), "... for out of the abundance of the heart the mouth speaketh" (Matthew 12:34), and "For out of the heart proceed evil thoughts, murders, adulteries, fornications, thefts, false witness, blasphemies: ..." (Matthew 15:19).

I believe it was Charles H. Spurgeon who said, "What's down in the well will come up in the bucket." What is in a person's heart will show in his deeds.

From these references, and there are more, it does seem that we can know something of what is in a person's heart. So believers are responsible to maintain the purity of the church as much as possible. The church is to be made up of regenerate people, as has been seen in the teaching of numerous passages of Scripture. Reasons as to why some believe otherwise have been seen to be completely bankrupt so far as any biblical basis is concerned and are seen to be the product of men's reasoning and incomplete understanding of the Scriptures.

RESULTS OF ROTTEN REASONING

The immediate result of the practice we have noticed is that the church came to be composed of a "mixt multitude," saved and unsaved. As Moses was leading the Israelites from Egypt to Canaan, "... the mixt multitude that was among them fell a lusting: and the children of Israel also wept again, and said, Who shall give us flesh to eat?" (Numbers 11:4). Notice, the true Israelites were soon affected by the mixt multitude. The same results were to be expected in the church when it was composed of saved and unsaved.

First, their moral standards were lowered. The church was no longer a special class of the elect. It included everyone. They were no longer a separate people because there was nothing to be separate from. It was all in the church. Instead of being different they came to be more and more like everyone else.

Even the leadership became corrupt, a fact that is well attested by many historians. The clergy used its position for self-aggrandizement. History records accounts of virtuous women who were sent to their death because they resisted the amorous advances of wicked priests.

Second, it would be only natural that doctrinal error would come in. A person who does not have the indwelling Holy Spirit as his teacher cannot understand the deep things of the Spirit of God. "But the natural man receiveth not the things of the Spirit of God: for they are foolishness unto him: neither can he know them, because they are spiritually discerned" (I Corinthians 2:14). Sure enough, in the course of time, there came such doctrinal errors as salvation by works, purgatory, soul sleep and prayers to saints and Mary; and on and on, ad infinitum.

With this as at least a partial explanation of the origin of false doctrine, perhaps we can see why there is so much of it that is being propagated today, even by people who give some evidence of salvation. Amazingly, false teachers are often much more dedicated than teachers of truth. Such doctrine, inculcated in the minds of men from their youth, is difficult to dislodge. Falsehood blinds; truth enlightens. However, it often seems that the false is the stronger of the two. It is certainly more deceptive.

Third, a combination of doctrinal error and practice was an inevitable result. Out of many, only one example will be cited. That one is "coercionism," the belief that a person could be made to believe if he were threatened with a horrible physical punishment should he not do so. It seems obvious that such a notion could come only from the minds of men who were not regenerate or, at best, had been greatly influenced by those who were not.

Last, but certainly not least, the unregenerate in the church would certainly result in spiritual deadness. The doctrinal system known as Calvinism has often been blamed for spiritual deadness in churches holding this view. While it is certainly true that Hyper-Calvinism can and does deaden individuals and churches spiritually, it is more than passing strange that churches of the reformed faith that are strongly Calvinistic also practice receiving unsaved people into their membership. Could this not just as well be the cause of deadness? It is certain that unregenerate people who have no spiritual life could do nothing to enhance the spirituality of a church. An unsaved person would care little, if anything, about the salvation of others and would have no concern about the biblical presentation of the gospel. He would certainly have no Spirit motivation for biblical worship.

REALIZING REALITY

It is certainly true that Baptists believe in a regenerate church membership. Some of them even know why others believe and practice otherwise. They also know some of the undesirable results of having unsaved people as members of the church. But how well do they measure up in practicing what they preach? Not too well, I'm afraid. Consider several reasons.

First, many church auditoriums are not large enough to accommodate all of the members should they happen to come on the same Sunday. Many would not have room for half of them. I recently read of a church that boasted a membership of well over fifty thousand. They had just built a new sanctuary that would seat only six thousand! Where are the rest?

Second, a church that I once pastored declined in membership from over five hundred to just about two hundred and fifty in four years. Yet the attendance almost doubled and the church became stronger in every way. Many of the members could not be found when I began, and when some of them were located their spiritual condition was disheartening to say the least.

Third, a growing number of Christians are complaining that they are not being spiritually fed. Yet, when able pastors begin to go deeper and provide spiritual food, the complaint of many is that he preaches over their heads. Could it be that these conditions exist because many to whom we minister have never really been born again? We are obligated to consider this possibility and then see if we cannot discover the reasons that it might be true. Let us look at some things that could result in our efforts bringing forth professors of salvation instead of possessors of salvation.

First, an emphasis on numbers instead of individuals could be a cause. Numbers are exciting, and it it easy, unwittingly, to begin to make numbers our goal while extolling the virtue and spirituality of reaching and winning souls. If numbers do become our priority, we will find that the next step is to use dubious, if not outright unbiblical, methods to get them to do something. Some seem to believe that if a person has "walked the aisle," for whatever purpose, he is saved. This just isn't so!

Second, because of a desire to reach great numbers, a trend toward "instant salvation" could well be one of the causes of unregenerate people going through all the motions but never really believing unto salvation. It is a common practice to pass out "gospills" which present the gospel in capsule form or to present brief, carefully contrived statements of the gospel that are designed to bring a person quickly to a decision. Could it be that because of our haste, we say to people, "... Believe on the Lord Jesus Christ, and thou shalt be saved, ..." (Acts 16:31); but the one addressed does not know who Jesus is, or what he is to believe, or why he should?

Third, perhaps we are in too big a hurry to get many "soul winners" into the field and do not adequately equip them for their task. The work of soul winning is not just giving a formulated plan and then getting them to "pray the prayer." It is true that anyone who "... shall call upon the name of the Lord shall be saved" (Romans 10:13). It is also true that Paul asked, "How then shall they call upon him in whom they have not believed? and how shall they believe in him of whom they have not heard . . . ?" (Romans 10:14). Calling without belief is a farce, and believing without having heard the facts is impossible. Perhaps we need to remember that our work is to be judged as to *what sort* it is, not *how much* it is (I Corinthians 3:13).

We would go a long way toward correcting this situation in which we find ourselves if, as we witness, we would patiently and thoroughly bear witness concerning the Person and Work of Jesus. Unsaved people need to be told that He is God! They need to know that He is holy, just, righteous, and eternal; and that He was tempted like as we are but without sin. They need to know that He was virgin born, that He died on the cross, thus becoming God's sin bearing lamb; and that He was buried, rose from the dead and ascended to the Father where He ever liveth to make intercession for His own. Then when we ask someone to believe on Him, they have something to believe. They will know who He is and what He did.

May we give careful thought to these things lest we be guilty of standing, doctrinally, for a truth but denying our own distinctive in practice.

BIBLIOGRAPHY

1. Kuiper, B. K., *The Church in History*. Grand Rapids, Michigan: Wm. B. Eerdmans Publishing Co., 1951. pp 68,69. Summary

2. Cairns, Earle E., *Christianity Through the Centuries*. Grand Rapids, Michigan: Zondervan Publishing House, 1954, 1967. p 134

3. Verduin, Leonard, *The Reformers and Their Stepchildren*. Grand Rapids, Michigan: Baker Book House, 1964. pp 30, 31

4. Adams, John Quincy, *Baptists, Thorough Reformers*. Rochester, New York: Backus Book Publishers, n.d. p 72

5. Ibid. p 73

6. Berkhof, Louis, *Systematic Theology*. Vol. II of 2 vols. Grand Rapids, Michigan: Wm. B. Eerdmans Publishing Co., 1938. p 239

7. Ibid. p 239

8. Ibid. p 239, 240

CHAPTER IV
SHALL WE GATHER AT THE RIVER?

Perhaps you remember this familiar song. For years it was the practice of Baptists to gather at the river for baptism; and, although this song has nothing at all to do with baptism, many thought it appropriate to sing at such a service. Baptism and rivers have long been associated, the idea being that much water is needed for biblical baptism. You see, Baptists believe in baptism by immersion and of believers only. Anything less than this does not constitute biblical baptism.

We have already seen that this is how Baptists got their name. Baptist means "baptizer." Somehow, the fact that they baptized by total immersion stood out in the minds of those who observed them. They saw that it was important to them. But just how important is this practice in the minds of Baptists? It is very important but not all important. By this we mean that it is not the most important thing in our doctrine or practice. For instance, the doctrine of *Salvation By Grace Through Faith* is much more important than that of *Baptism By Immersion* Of Believers. The first has to do with salvation and affects a person's eternal destiny, but the second has to do with a person's obedience and affects him in the area of rewards. Baptism is essential, not to a person's salvation but to obedience.

Some, who were Baptists, have taken the importance of baptism to the extreme and have taught that it is essential to salvation. Alexander Campbell was one of them, and the sect known as the Campbellites or Disciples of Christ was started because of his teaching. However, when anyone teaches that it is necessary to be baptized in order to be saved, he soon finds that he cannot teach that salvation is by grace since baptism is a work, and salvation by grace is not obtained "... by works of righteousness which we have done, ..." (Titus 3:5). Further, one false doctrine leads to another, and it follows logically that if a person can be saved by doing something, he can also be lost by doing, or not doing, something. And from that point there is no end to the false teachings that can be spawned, all from one wrong conclusion.

As we proceed, always keep in mind that Baptists baptize as a matter of obedience, not as a means of salvation. They are baptized because they have been saved, not in order to be saved. But they do believe that being baptized biblically is very important. Baptism is not optional for Christians; we do not have the right to choose to be or not to be baptized. Neither do we have the right to choose the method that suits us best. The proper mode is clearly delineated in the Bible, and it is up to us to find it and use it.

Yet, it is difficult for some to see that baptism is all that important, especially since it has nothing to do with salvation. However, historically Baptists have considered this distinctive important enough to die for. Much, if not most, of the persecution of our predecessors was caused by their belief and practice in this area and by other practices, such as rebaptism, that partly grew out of this doctrine. So, while Baptists have been willing to die for this belief, their adversaries have been more than willing for them to die!

Our discussion that will follow immediately will deal with two questions; (1) Why do others baptize any other way, and (2) Why do Baptists baptize by immersion? In doing this we shall consider statements from Louis Berkhof, a theologian of the reformed faith. His views are quite representative of those who do not wish to immerse. As I recall, others who have written more recently have used many of the same arguments that Berkhof uses, thus following the same party line. But Berkhof's arguments can be ably answered. Basically, he offers three arguments for baptizing by methods other than immersion: (1) the significance of baptism, (2) the meaning of the Greek word that is translated "baptize", and (3) that three thousand would have been too many to baptize in one day if they were immersed.

First, consider his belief about the symbolic significance of baptism. He writes,

> Reformed theology has an entirely different view [from Baptists] of the essential thing in the symbolism of baptism. It finds this in the idea of purification.... Moreover, Scripture makes it abundantly clear that baptism symbolizes spiritual cleansing or purification,....
>
> ... The generally prevailing opinion outside of Baptist circles is that as long as the fundamental idea, namely, that of purification, finds expression in the rite, the mode of baptism is quite immaterial. It may be administered by immersion, by pouring or effusion, or by sprinkling....[1]

I suppose, in case of an emergency, a damp cloth would be sufficient as long as it symbolized purification in some way.

Certainly, no one could disagree with the belief that baptism does signify purification, cleansing, or washing with reference to sins. However, while pouring or sprinkling water upon someone would signify this, albeit weakly, immersion would signify it more clearly. What better way is there to signify cleansing or washing than by total immersion in water?

But Scripture reveals other things that baptism signifies; and these can be shown only by immersion, not by sprinkling or pouring. Consider first that the believer is counted by God to be dead, buried, and risen with Jesus. Baptists believe there is strong scriptural evidence that baptism should picture this. Paul wrote of believers, "For ye are dead, and your life is hid with Christ in God" (Colossians 3:3). In another place he continues this thought by writing, "Therefore we are buried with him by baptism into death: that like as Christ was raised up from the dead by the glory of the Father, even so we also should walk in newness of life" (Romans 6:4). The idea of baptism as a burial is seen further in these words, "Buried with him in baptism, wherein also ye are risen with him through the faith of the operation of God, who hath raised him from the dead" (Colossians 2:12).

Therefore, baptism signifies that one who is saved has, in God's sight, died with Christ, been buried with Him, and has risen with Him. This can be shown, symbolically, by being buried beneath the water and then being raised up from under the water. It cannot be shown, to any degree, by having water poured or sprinkled upon a person.

There is more. Scripture states, "Therefore if any man be in Christ, he is a new creature: old things are passed away; behold, all things are become new" (II Corinthians 5:17). There is no better way to symbolize this than by rising from a burial in a watery grave to walk in newness of life.

In summary, while the washing or cleansing aspect of baptism can be shown better by immersion than by sprinkling or pouring, the death, burial, and resurrection aspect cannot be pictured at all by either of these last two methods. It must be done by baptizing by immersion. While it might be disputed which of these significations is the primary one, there can be no doubt that they are both present in Scripture. That being true, is it not more logical to use the method of baptism that pictures both of them rather than a method that, at best, can picture only one of them?

Second, Berkhof appeals to a supposed meaning of the Greek word that is translated by the English word, "baptize." In introducing this subject, however, he deals briefly with biblical examples of baptism. Says he, "Neither do the Biblical examples of baptism stress any particular mode."[2] Now I realize that scholars say there are so many different meanings to some prepositions in the Greek language that we cannot be sure if the Greek preposition, *eis*, means into or unto. Therefore, we cannot be sure if John and Jesus or Philip and the eunuch went down *into* the water or down *unto* the water. But there are several graphic descriptions of baptisms that offer us some help. Consider one of them.

Remember, after Philip had preached Jesus to the eunuch, the eunuch said, "... See, here is water; what doth hinder me to be baptized?" (Acts 8:36). After Philip was satisfied that the eunuch believed, "... he commanded the chariot to stand still: and they went down *both* into the water, *both* Philip and the eunuch; and he baptized him" (Acts 8:38). Those who like to play with prepositions say this could read, "they went down to the water" and "they came up from the edge of the water." However, this effort would not have been necessary if Philip was only going to sprinkle a few drops of water on the eunuch. Certainly there was enough water in the chariot to do this. Yet, they made their way from the chariot to the water that had attracted the eunuch's attention. Why? Because they were going to go "... down into the water, both Philip and the eunuch ...." Why this need? This action on their part was taken so the eunuch could be baptized by immersion. This is the only thing that makes sense; therefore, this example is a clear case of baptism by immersion. The circumstances demand this conclusion!

Let us return to the meaning of the word that is translated "baptize." Bapto, from which baptizo is derived, is the word and of it Berkhof writes,

> ... Baptists were very confident at one time that this verb means only "to dip"; but many of them changed their mind since Dr. Carson, one of their greatest authorities, came to the conclusion that it also has a secondary meaning, namely, "to dye," so that it came to mean "to dye by dipping," and even "to dye in any manner," ....[3]

Notice, the secondary meaning is "to dye." Then the tertiary meaning is to "dye by dipping." (Note: Tertiary is to three what secondary is to two and primary is to one.) What better way is there to dye a piece of cloth than to dip or immerse the cloth in water containing dye? But Berkhof does not stop here. He proceeds to a fourth-hand meaning and says it came to mean "... even 'to dye in any manner,' thus ceasing to be modal."[4] Evidently this guy just doesn't want to get wet!

Now Berkhof has a question. Was baptizo derived from bapto in its primary meaning, or from bapto in its secondary meaning? Either of these meanings would present a strong case for immersion, so Berkhof seems to want to accept the fourth-hand meaning as the one he will go by, But is this acceptable? Dr. J. L. Dagg, an outstanding scholar of the last century, gives us this rule:

> In the ordinary process of translating the writings of a Greek author, when we wish to ascertain the meaning of some word that he uses, we satisfy ourselves, for the most part, by consulting a Greek lexicon.
> The laws of interpretation require us to take the primary signification of words, unless there be something in the context, or nature of the subject, inconsistent with this signification. As there is no such difficulty in the present instance, our first decision, if we follow the lexicons, must be in favor of the sense to *immerse*.[5] (Emphasis is his.)

Dr. Carson follows this rule, as is shown by his statement that "... it is derived from bapto in the sense of 'to dip.' ... 'My position is that it always signifies to dip, never expressing anything but mode.' "[6]

It is interesting that scholars of other denominations than Baptists seem to be pretty much in agreement that the primary meaning of the word "baptizo" is to immerse. Yet they appeal to the secondary and tertiary meanings of the word; and as we have seen, some even go further in an attempt to justify their practice of sprinkling or pouring.

Next, Berkhof tries to cast doubt on the practice of immersion by asking,

> ... Did John dip the multitudes that flocked unto him at the river Jordan; and did the apostles dip the five [sic] thousand that were converted on the day of Pentecost?[7]

The idea is that it would have taken too much time to immerse so great a number of converts. Yet, it seems to me that in order for the administrator of the ordinance to give proper solemnity to the occasion it would take quite some time even by sprinkling. Of course, he could just throw a bucket of water over all of them at once.

However, that three thousand could be baptized in one day by immersion is shown by Strong. He argues,

> ... There was no difficulty in baptizing three thousand in one day; for, in the time of Chrysostom, when all candidates of the year were baptized in a single day, three thousand were once baptized; and, on July 3, 1878, 2222 ... Christians were baptized by two administrators in nine hours.... The same two men did not baptize all the time. There were six men engaged in baptizing, but never more than two at the same time.[8]

Church historian, Thomas Armitage tells of three thousand being immersed in one day and evidently by one man. He wrote of a place that was a natural baptistery

> ... where Paulinus administered Christian immersion. The vicar of Harbottle has caused a crucifix to be erected in the center, with the following inscription: 'In this place Paulinus the bishop baptized three thousand Northumbrians, Easter 627.'[9]

Notice that the method used was immersion according to Armitage. No pun is intended, but Berkhof's arguments simply do not hold water.

There is really no reason to go further to establish the biblical practice of immersion. John Quincy Adams believed that if the word "baptizo" had been translated instead of being transliterated the word "immerse" would have been used instead of the word "baptize." Giving a Greek word an English spelling tells us nothing about the real meaning.

There is one other interesting item that points to the practice of immersion, and that is the existence of baptisteries down through the centuries that are of such a construction that they would make no sense unless they were used for immersion. Armitage gives pictures of a number of them.

During a tour of Israel in 1977, I visited the ruins of the settlement where the Essenes had lived in the first century A.D. The Essenes practiced numerous washings or baptisms. They were, of course, Jews and not Christians. Their method of baptism was immersion, however. This is shown by a tank that has been discovered there that greatly resembles a modern baptistery, steps and all. Their method in the first century A.D. must have been immersion. There is no reason to believe that the baptism of John, or of Jesus, was anything else.

BELIEVERS' BAPTISM

In the last chapter we discussed the belief of Baptists concerning a regenerate church membership. This, of course, implies a belief in believers' baptism, i.e., that only those who believe in Jesus as Saviour and Lord and are, therefore, regenerate are proper subjects for baptism. Those who do not so believe are not scripturally baptized although they have gone through the form and ceremony of baptism by immersion. While the biblical reasons for this have been covered somewhat already, we do need to consider several direct reasons for our belief, since the results of this doctrine have had such a profound effect on Baptist life.

First, the order of the Great Commission places baptism after belief. Jesus commanded His disciples, "Go ye therefore, and teach all nations, [i.e., make disciples] baptizing them in the name of the Father, and of the Son, and of the Holy Ghost: Teaching them to observe all things whatsoever I have commanded you: . . ." (Matthew 28:19-20). Notice, first make disciples, then baptize them; and, last of all, teach them. This definitely excludes infants from baptism; it also excludes anyone of whatever age who has not become a disciple.

Second, consider the case of the Ethiopian eunuch. After he had heard the gospel from Philip he said, "... See, here is water; what doth hinder me to be baptized?" (Acts 8:36). Philip's answer was, "... If thou believest with all thine heart, thou mayest ..." (Acts 8:37). It is obvious; belief was necessary before baptism! Philip definitely believed in and practiced believers' baptism.

The last reason that we shall consider is that baptism of one who does not believe is a violation of the symbolic significance of the ordinance. We have just seen that water baptism pictures the death, burial, and resurrection of the one being baptized. But if that one has not believed, he has not been counted by God to be dead with Christ. He is still dead in trespasses and sins. He has experienced no resurrection to walk in newness of life. He is still walking "... according to the course of this world, according to the prince of the power of the air, the spirit that now worketh in the children of disobedience: ..." (Ephesians 2:2). For him, baptism would mean nothing because nothing about him has changed. He is not a new creature in Christ. Actually, to ascribe a biblical meaning to the baptism of such a person would be near blasphemy. This would be true even if cleansing or purification were the only thing that baptism signified.

ORIGIN OF ANABAPTISTS

Because of what Baptists believed concerning this matter a practice emerged of baptizing new believers who had been baptized as infants or before they were saved. Pedobaptists called this rebaptism and named the ones who did it Anabaptists or Rebaptizers. This practice and name surfaced during the period of the Reformation, but that was not the beginning of it. It is believed by reputable historians to have originated as early as the coming of the Constantinian State-Church and the infant baptism, etc., that grew out of it. Actually, it happened

A PEOPLE FOR HIS NAME

much earlier, as we shall see presently.

It should also be noted that those who practiced this did not consider it to be rebaptism. They did not believe that those whom they baptized had been baptized in the first place. They had only taken part in a ceremony that involved water in one form or another. This was not scriptural baptism!

An example of rebaptizing some who had evidently not believed, savingly, on Jesus is found in Acts 19:1-7. The apostle Paul was the rebaptizer, or Anabaptist, in this case. When he was in Ephesus he found certain disciples who had not received the Holy Spirit. In fact, they had not heard that there was such a person. Upon questioning them, Paul found that they had been baptized with John's baptism. He then explained that John's was a baptism of repentance but that he had preached that they should believe on one who was to come after him, that is, on Christ Jesus. Apparently they had not done this. Perhaps they had not heard the gospel, that Jesus had died, been buried, and had risen again. When they heard this (evidently with approval) they were baptized, by Paul or someone in his party, in the name of the Lord Jesus. This is a clear-cut case of rebaptizing, making Paul the first Anabaptist of whom we have any record.

A COLLISION COURSE

We are now beginning to see something of how many of the Baptist distinctives are interrelated. Some of them grew out of others in such a way that to believe one demanded belief in one or more of the others. Believing as they did, the Baptists soon found themselves on a collision course with others who claimed to be Christians. This set the stage for some of the bloodiest chapters in church history as well as for the emergence of more Baptist distinctives.

Our predecessors believed in the Bible as their only sufficient authority; others did not. They believed in a regenerate church membership; others did not. They believed in believers' baptism; others baptized unregenerate folks. They rejected infant baptism; others practiced it. They believed that baptism was to be by total immersion; others believed sprinkling or pouring to be just as good. It is easy to see how this set them at odds with just about everyone else in Christendom.

SUFFERING SAINTS

Unfortunately, this was not at a time when people were willing to live and let live, not even those claiming to be Christians. In a previous chapter we noticed the practice of coercing people to become church members and to believe a certain way. This coercion took many forms, among which were confiscation of property, banishment, torture by the most horrible methods and death in the most horrendous ways. This was done by the church that was in power before the Reformation and, later, by the Reformers themselves. Those holding our distinctives suffered under both.

It is not within the scope of this work to give complete treatment to the subject of persecution and suffering that has been caused by these differences. The reader is urged to avail himself of books that do cover this subject and read for himself. It is not beyond the realm of possibility or even probability that Christians will again be called upon to suffer for their faith, even in Christian America.

Almost any good church history will relate some of this suffering. *Fox's Book of Martyrs* is a classic and documents many incidents of martyrdom. I have a rare two-volume set, *The Israel of the Alps*, which tells of the awful persecution of the Vaudois, the Waldenses, by the Roman Catholic Church. Of course, the Church used the civil authorities to do the actual work. I understand these two volumes have been reprinted. And, of course, there are many others.

The means of torture and punishment that were used by the enemies of the Anabaptists in an effort to get them to recant were many. Beheading, which is self-explanatory, was one of them. During the Dark Ages and the Reformation as well, death by being burned at the stake was common. Often the sentence was that the victim was to be burned by a slow fire, using either green or wet wood. At times, friends of the victim would hang a bag of explosive gun powder around the victim's neck in order to shorten the time of his misery. The rack was used, a device upon which the victim was fastened so he could be stretched until his joints were separated from their sockets. Even their imprisonment was unbelievably unbearable and inhuman. Armitage described that of Balthazar Hubmeyer as being in a place where

> ... no light of sun or moon penetrated, where bread and water were the only nourishment, and these could not be taken for days together, on account of the sickening odors of the place; where the living were shut up with the dead, with no hope of escape but in death or recantation....[10]

Such things as this are unbelievable in our day, but they are well documented by many reputable historians.

Another means of death was deviously devised, evidently especially for the Anabaptists, that being death by drowning! Out of many who sealed their faith by martyrdom in this manner we will detail only one. He was Felix Mantz (or Manz; the spelling varies with different writers), a native of Zurich, Switzerland, and a noble Baptist leader according to Armitage.

Mantz held views about baptism with which the Reformers did not agree. One of his chief adversaries was Ulrich Zwingli, one of the most notable of the Swiss Reformers. Mantz preached that infants should not be baptized, that only the regenerate should hold church membership, that those who were baptized as infants or before salvation should be baptized after they were saved, and that civil powers should have no control over men in spiritual matters. He was arrested and stayed in prison for a long time, where he suffered much and lived on bread and water. He was offered his release from prison if he would stop baptizing. He managed to escape along with about twenty others but was later arrested and finally sentenced to death. The day of his execution was to be January 5, 1527. Armitage gives the following account:

> ... His sentence gave him over to the executioner, who put him into a boat, bound his hands over his knees, put a block between his arms and legs, [and] threw him into the water to drown, ... He was led on the day of his slaughter from the Wellenburg, the heretics' tower, through the fish-market and shambles to a boat, preaching to the people as he went. A Reformed pastor at his side sought to silence him, but his faithful brother and his old mother brushed away their tears and exhorted him to suffer firmly for Jesus' sake. The executioner put the black cap on his head, bound him to a hurdle and threw him into Lake Zurich, as he cried, with Jesus, "Into thy hands I commend my spirit!"[11]

Others were put to death in the same manner, some being bound together with chains in such a way that when one was pushed from the boat, he would pull the next into the water after him, and so on until they all perished. Remember, this was done with the approval of Zwingli and other Reformers. There is evidence that he was the outright instigator of it, as we shall have occasion to see a little later. How strange that the Reformers who had suffered severely at the hands of the Catholic Church now became the persecutors. We shall see later that this was so because they retained much of the philosophy that the Catholic Church had held.

UNBAPTIZED BAPTISTS?

A question has arisen about the way in which Felix Mantz was baptized. Was it by immersion? Was this the reason he was sentenced to death by drowning? It should be noted that baptism by immersion was not the only reason Baptists were hated. Other reasons were their refusal to have their infants baptized; their practice of rebaptizing, on a confession of faith, those who had been sprinkled as infants; and their refusal to admit the rule of the state over the church. But the question of the method of the baptism of Mantz and others about that time provides an interesting study.

Some Baptists believe immersion was not the method. Benson says, "These Anabaptists at this stage [1525, two years before Mantz was drowned] did not practice immersion, and so were not really Baptists."[12] After having done research in England for three months, William Heth Whitsitt, president of Southern Baptist Seminary in Louisville, Kentucky, in the latter part of the nineteenth century, published an article in *Johnson's Universal Cyclopedia* in which he wrote, "...Roger Williams was probably baptized by sprinkling rather than by immersion and that immersion of believers among English Baptists was 'invented' by Edward Barber in 1641."[13] So great was the controversy over this that Whitsitt resigned as president of the seminary, the resignation to take effect at the close of the session of 1898-1899.

The venerable Baptist historian, John T. Christian, gives documented evidence to the contrary, however. He claims,

> The practice of immersion was universal in the reign of Henry VIII [1509-1547]. It was the form of baptism of all parties and there is no known testimony to the contrary. The Church of England practiced immersion. The Catholics practiced immersion. The Baptists practiced immersion.[14]

If this is true, we must conclude that Whitsitt was wrong and that English Baptists who were the recipients of severe persecution were punished because of the other reasons mentioned above, not just because they immersed.

But was Felix Mantz immersed? Remember, Mantz lived in Switzerland, not England. Christian quotes an anonymous Moravian chronicle which claims that Conrad Grebel, a close associate of Mantz, baptized George Jacob Blaurock when he fell upon his knees in a church meeting. This seems to imply sprinkling or pouring. Armitage says he poured water on his head. The same chronicle says of Mantz's baptizing John Brubach that, "He then took a dipper of water and baptized him...." However, Christian contends,

> If the events described above took place, of which there is much doubt, it was at the time Grebel had first broken with Zwingli, and was still a Presbyterian, and Blaurock had just come from the Roman Catholic Church, and before either of them had embraced Baptist views....[15]

This is quite possible. No one contends that those in the past came to all of the Baptist views in one fell swoop.

However, Christian contends that the chronicle is spurious. To conserve space, the following summary of his reasons is offered.

> It is anonymous; no author who quotes from it claims to have seen it. No date or page is ever given. The language is that of Pedobaptists not the Anabaptists of that time. It is contrary to the known fact that Grebel, a few days later, was in the practice of dipping, and that Manz practiced dipping.[16]

As early as March 1525, Conrad Grebel baptized by dipping. It is unreasonable to assume that his close associate, Felix Mantz, would not have held the same view by the time he was executed by drowning, January 5, 1527.

Last of all, let us consult our friend, Verduin. Remember he is of the Reformed Faith and as such would adhere to sprinkling or effusion, not immersion. He reasons,

> Zwingli's "most unkindest cut of all" occurred when he said, "Let him who talks about 'going under' go under [the water]!" It may

well have been this unkind word that inspired men to truss up Felix Manz so that he could not swim, and to send him thus bound to the bottom of the Limmat! Manz had talked about "going under" in baptism; well then let him have his fill of it! ...[17]

To paraphrase Zwingli's words, let the punishment fit the crime. Verduin has reasoned correctly. The execution of Mantz in this manner would make no sense at all if he did not believe in and practice baptism by immersion. Talk about total immersion, Zwingli went from the sublime to the ridiculous in this matter. What began as an issue of total immersion ended, for Mantz, as a matter of terminal submersion.

BIBLIOGRAPHY

1. Berkhof, Louis, *Systematic Theology*. Vol. II of 2 vols. Grand Rapids, Michigan: Wm. B. Eerdmans Publishing Co., 1938, pp 236, 237

2. Ibid., p 237

3. Ibid., p 237

4. Ibid., p 237

5. Dagg, John L., *Manual of Theology and Church Order*. Harrisonburg, Virginia: Gano Books, 1982 2nd Part, pp 21, 22

6. Berkhof, Ibid., pp 237, 238

7. Ibid., p 238

8. Strong, *Systematic Theology*. Vol. III of 3 vols. Philadelphia, Pennsylvania: The Judson Press, 1909. p 934

9. Armitage, Thomas, *History of the Baptists*. New York, New York: Bryan, Taylor & Co., 1890. p 254

10. Ibid., p 338

11. Ibid., p 335

12. Benson, John L., *The Dynamic People Called Baptists*. Denver, Colorado: Accent Micro-Books; 1974. p 27

13. Mueller, William A., *A History of Southern Baptist Theological Seminary.* Nashville, Tennessee: Broadman Press, 1959. p 155

14. Christian, John T., *A History of the Baptists.* Vol. I of 2 vols. Nashville, Tennessee: Broadman Press, 1928. P 196

15. Ibid., pp 116,117

16. Ibid., p 117

17. Verduin, Leonard, *The Reformers and Their Stepchildren.* Grand Rapids, Michigan: Baker Book House, 1980. p 217

CHAPTER V
ROCK-A-BYE-BABY

Sometime between 1846 and 1903 Charles Dupee Blake penned the following lines,

Rock-a-bye-baby on the tree top,
When the wind blows the cradle will rock,
When the bough breaks the cradle will fall,
And down will come baby, cradle and all.

Somehow I can't help wondering how a baby could possibly find himself in such a hapless situation, or why any responsible parent would place an infant in such a precarious position. However, history records many instances of parents taking what appears to be unfair advantage of their children. In bygone days parents sometimes offered their children as burnt sacrifices in order to appease heathen gods or to gain favor from them. The Old Testament tells of times when Israelites "... built the high places of Tophet, which is in the valley of the sons of Hinnom, to burn their sons and their daughters in the fire; ..." (Jeremiah 7:31). Comparatively recent archaeological discoveries in Carthage have revealed urns filled with the skeletal remains of small infants that have evidently been offered in such ceremonial sacrifices.

While not as detrimental to their physical well being, parents have more recently subjected their infants to certain religious rites in which these children could have no conscious part. And while, in most cases, it would not be physically damaging, it will be shown that it can and will be used later in life to hinder their freedom of conscience in matters pertaining to religion. The practice to which I refer is infant baptism, a practice that is performed long before the child has reached the age of accountability or the years of discretion.

Those who practice infant baptism are called Pedobaptists. The image we usually have of the baptismal ceremony which they perform is of a priest, preacher, or whoever sprinkling a few drops of water on a fairly young baby. However, although this is the method used in most cases now, it has not always been so. There are numerous references to times in the past when children were baptized by dipping. At one time trine immersion of infants was practiced. Some said that if the child was in too weak a condition he could be baptized by having water sprinkled or poured on him while still in his clothes. Some dissented, however. Tyndale (Martyred in 1536) had written,

> If aught be left out, or if the child be not altogether dipped in water, or if, because the child is sick, the priest dare not plunge it into the water, but pour water upon its head, — How tremble they . . . . Hath it full Christendom? They believe verily, that the child is not christened.[1]

Although the biblical method of baptism by immersion has been clearly seen in the previous chapter, that is not the question here. Baptists believe that infants should not be baptized regardless of the method. What grounds do they have for such a belief, and why do others believe in such a practice as this? In answering these questions, we shall see that more space is required to show why some do than to show why Baptists do not. Yet, a good bit of time and space will be required to answer the false conclusions that led to a belief in the necessity of infant baptism.

Obviously, a basic cause of this practice is a belief that an infant who dies unbaptized is lost. Recently, at the close of a Sunday morning worship service, I was approached by a man and two of his children, one about three years of age. He said that he had come to see about getting them baptized. Upon being questioned as to why he wanted them baptized he replied that he felt that if they died they would have a better chance of salvation than if they were not baptized. This notion, of course, was the product of two false beliefs: first, that those who die before reaching the years of discretion are lost and, second, that baptism has some power to convey salvation in such a situation. As far as I can see these two ideas would have to be present in the thought of any one who considered baptism of infants of any great importance. But are these two beliefs correct? Actually, if the first (that those who die before reaching the years of discretion are lost) is false, then the second is irrelevant in this case.

Unfortunately, Scripture does not provide many answers to this question, but it does provide enough that we can ascertain the truth. When David's baby that Bathsheba had borne him died, David said, "... Can I bring him back again? I shall go to him, but he shall not return to me" (II Samuel 12:23). This shows that David had a belief in life after death and that he would, in that life, be in the same place as his departed baby. This leaves no doubt; David believed this child was saved.

However, this baby was not saved just because he was a baby. He had a sin nature just like everyone else. Scripture says of babies, "The wicked are estranged from the womb: they go astray as soon as they be born, speaking lies" (Psalm 58:3). There is no record that would indicate that he was saved because of any ceremony that was performed on his behalf, nor is there any prescription in the Bible for any such salvatory ceremony. We must believe, then, that since there is no way of salvation but Jesus, God, in some way not understood by us, saved this child and all others by His Grace.

Another passage of Scripture that is often used in attempting to answer the question of the salvation of infants is found in three of the Gospels. We shall consider only one of them since they are all substantially the same.

> And they brought young children to him, that he should touch them: and his disciples rebuked those that brought them. But when Jesus saw it, he was much displeased, and said unto them, Suffer

A PEOPLE FOR HIS NAME

the little children to come unto me, and forbid them not: for of such is the kingdom of God.... And he took them up in his arms, put his hands upon them, and blessed them (Mark 10:13-16).

Bengel is quoted as saying, "He had no children that He might adopt all children." Whether this is true or not I cannot say. It does seem that Jesus would have said so if there were something that these children were capable of doing and that they needed to do but had not done. In this case He blessed them, but there was no action on their part to bring forth the blessing except that they had the characteristics of little children. Whether they were saved or not, I cannot say. It is noteworthy that Jesus did not say anything about the necessity of getting them baptized.

Admittedly, this does not give us much Scripture upon which to base any teaching of the salvation of infants; but it is a great deal more than those who teach infant baptism have to prove their case since there is none, as they readily admit. But why does it matter to parents if their infants are regenerate or not? Of course, it is only natural that they would be concerned as to the eternal destiny of their little ones. It would be a great comfort to know that such a one was safe with Jesus. I believe we can take comfort in the Scripture that we have considered and believe this is true. But suppose we were to conclude that infants are not saved? Biblically, there is nothing that could be done about it. There is only one way of salvation revealed in the Bible, that being Jesus. However, it is not possible to preach Him to a baby who has no understanding of language. Further, Jesus must be received by faith, and an infant cannot do that. What hope is there? Either God must save this one or he will not be saved. I believe it is only reasonable to believe that God will do just that. Frankly, I would believe this even if there were not so much as one passage of Scripture to indicate it. It is consistent with God's nature.

Evidently, those who believe in infant baptism are not satisfied that this matter can be left solely in God's care. Just as evidently, they believe that baptism has some power to save. However, even those who believe in baptismal regeneration would require that baptism be administered along with faith of some sort. But infants are not able to believe; so a practice of faith by proxy, or letting the parents' faith count for the child's faith, came into being. So, those who believed this way began to search for some Bible justification for what they were doing; and their search led them, New Testament Christians, to the Old Testament! Here again we find the result of failing to discern the dispensational difference between the people of God in the Old Testament and His people in the New Testament. Let us consider some of their reasoning.

THE SOUND OF SILENCE

For a long time Baptists have argued against infant baptism on the ground that it is nowhere commanded in Scripture. Pedobaptists agree that it is not commanded in the New Testament, but then proceed with the following argument which probably originated with Zwingli. He said, "The New Testament does not command the baptism of infants, neither does it forbid it; therefore we must look to the Old Testament for an analogy that will clear up the matter."[2] So, if what you want to do cannot be found in the New Testament, look in the Old Testament; and if you can't find any direct doctrine an analogy will do. This appears to be pretty much a case of deciding what you are going to believe and practice beforehand and then searching the Scriptures for justification for it. However, as we have already seen, this bypasses the authority of Scripture and cannot help but lead to error, since it makes man the final authority.

Before we consider the Old Testament analogy to which Zwingli appealed, let us look at his statement that "The New Testament does not command the baptism of infants, neither does it forbid it; . . . ."[3] This same line of reasoning is followed by more contemporary writers.

Berkhof, replying to the argument that there is no explicit command in Scripture that children must be baptized, reasons, "May not the silence of Scripture be construed as an argument for rather than against infant baptism? . . . Does the Bible anywhere command the exclusion of children from baptism; . . . ?"[4] This is nothing but an argument based on silence and in matters as important as this can only lead to erroneous conclusions. Yet, many present day Pedobaptist writers still use this argument to justify their practice. A number of Baptists have seen this error and have suggested that they are "baptizing in obedience to the silence of the New Testament."

Berkhof, in order to justify the practice of infant baptism in spite of the silence of Scripture, charges Baptists with inconsistency since they do things that are not commanded in Scripture. As an example, he says the Bible does not say that women should partake of the Lord's Supper; yet, this is Baptist practice. His argument is fallacious. There is an obvious New Testament reason why women who are regenerate should eat the Lord's Supper ". . . in remembrance of me" (I Corinthians 11:24). Further, Berkhof errs in this charge unless he is able to show that the Corinthian Church was composed only of males; which, of course, he cannot do. Paul's salutatory address to the Corinthian Church is, "Unto the church of God which is at Corinth, to them that are sanctified in Christ Jesus, called to be saints, with all that in every place call upon the name of Jesus Christ our Lord, both theirs and ours: . . ." (I Corinthians 1:2). That this salutation included women is a fact that we do not have to assume. There are too many statements made directly to women for us to have the least doubt about this. For instance, "Nevertheless, to avoid fornication, let every man have his own wife, and let every woman have her own husband" (I Corinthians 7:2). See also verses three and four. Then notice that chapter eleven of this same book gives instructions to women concerning their covering when they pray; and in a later chapter we read, "Let your women keep silence in the churches: for it is not permitted unto them to speak; . . ." (I Corinthians 14:34). Therefore, we conclude that there were women in the Corinthian congregation; and they were included in Paul's salutation and in the address of the letter. They were included in the instructions concerning the meaning and observance of the Lord's Supper.

It may be objected that this passage uses the words "men" and "brethren" when giving instructions for self examination, etc., before taking the supper. While this is true, it is in keeping with New Testament custom of addressing men alone when the message includes women as well. However, there is no such custom of doing this when the message or instructions included infants. Whatever inconsistency exists in this matter is only in Berkhof's mind.

However, speaking of inconsistencies, Armitage has the following concerning Zwingli and infant baptism.

> ... Playing fast and loose with the New Testament himself, and baptizing children in obedience to the "silence" of the New Testament, still he demanded of the Baptists a positive injunction of Christ for baptizing on a confession of him those who had been christened as babes. So he could stand coolly by and see the Baptists drowned, but surely not because the New Testament was silent on the subject of drowning Baptists. If its silence gave consent to the baptism of infants, certainly it did not render the legal murder of Baptists holy. Well might he admit that "nothing cost him so much sweat as his controversy with the Baptists."[5]

Baptists readily admit that there are many things that Baptists practice about which the New Testament is silent, and it is not wrong to do them. For instance, the New Testament says nothing about the use of pianos or organs or hymn books and tuning forks. It says nothing about the use of church pews or church buildings as we have today. Yet Baptists use all of these. They are a means to accomplish something that we are commanded, i.e., "Speaking to yourselves in psalms and hymns and spiritual songs, singing and making melody in your heart to the Lord; ..." (Ephesians 5:19) and, "Not forsaking the assembling of ourselves together, ..." (Hebrews 10:25). However, there is no such New Testament command that is accomplished by baptizing infants.

Baptists have, especially in recent times, had dedication services for infants. The New Testament does not command this for Christians, but there is nothing wrong with such a practice as long as it is well understood that it is just that and nothing more. It should be well explained that it has nothing to do with salvation, it does not admit the child to church membership, and it is not done in obedience to any biblical command. Perhaps there would not be anything wrong with throwing a few drops of water on the baby as long as there was no claim that it was biblical baptism, that it accomplished something spiritually for the child that could be done in no other way, or that it fulfilled God's command in some way. Of course, there would be no reason for doing such a thing either; and I certainly would not recommend it. Biblically, the service of the church is revealed as being utterly simple. There is no need to do anything that is not commanded unless it can be used to accomplish something for which there is an explicit command in the New Testament.

Going further with their argument from silence, Pedobaptists claim that infants must have been baptized in such cases as that of the Philippian jailor. Paul said to him, "... Believe on the Lord Jesus Christ, and thou shalt be saved, *and thy house*" (Acts 16:31). We are told further, "And he took them the same hour of the night, and washed their stripes; and was baptized, *he and all his*, straightway" (v 33). Pedobaptists claim the words, "*and thy house*" and "*he and all his*" must have included infants; although, admittedly, it does not say so. Baptists are willing to admit the possibility that there were infants in this house. But a close perusal of the passage does not warrant the belief that they were baptized that night. Consider several reasons.

First, the phrases are limited by the local context if it is considered logically. The first is very simple. If the jailor believed on the Lord Jesus Christ he would be saved. This promise also applied to his house. If those of his house believed they would be saved; if some of them did not believe they would not be saved. The jailor's faith was not sufficient to save his wife, adult children, or adult servants. Only personal faith would avail for them. So unless they all believed they would not all be saved. This limits the phrase, *"and thy house,"* so that it includes only those of his house who believed. This rules out babies. It must also be understood in this way in the following verses where it or its equivalent is used.

Consider also that before the baptismal service Paul ". . . spake unto him the word of the Lord, and to *all that were in his house"* (v 32). Now imagine this scene. The hour is sometime between midnight and the break of day. All the infants are awakened and taken from their beds so Paul can speak the Word to "all that were in his house." Then, sometime in the wee hours of the morning, these babies, along with believing adults, were baptized. Are these little ones now to be returned to their beds so they can continue their peaceful slumber? No! Meat must be set before Paul and his party; and the jailor is going to spend some time rejoicing and believing, "with all his house," babies and all. Several stanzas of Rock-A-Bye-Baby will need to be sung before this household is back to normal.

In the second place, to believe that these phrases teach that infants who were in the house were baptized is contrary to the general context of the New Testament. We have already seen that salvation is by grace through faith, personal faith; and baptism is to be preceded by regeneration according to New Testament Scripture. In interpreting Scripture we dare not make an individual passage contradict the overall teaching of the Bible.

OLD TESTAMENT TEACHING FOR NEW TESTAMENT PRACTICE

We now turn with the Pedobaptists to the Old Testament to see where, in its pages, they are going to find authority for the baptism of infants; and they find it based on the covenant God made with Abraham. Building upon this concept, Berkhof presents four arguments for his New Testament practice of infant baptism.

> (1) The covenant made with Abraham was primarily a spiritual covenant, though it also had a national aspect, and of this spiritual covenant circumcision was a sign and seal . . . .
>
> (2) This covenant is still in force and is essentially identical with the "new covenant" of the present dispensation . . . .
>
> (3) By the appointment of God infants shared in the benefits of the covenant, and therefore received circumcision as a sign and seal . . . . This national idea is naturally very prominent in the Old Testament, but it is carried right over into the New Testament, . . . we would hardly expect the privileges of such children to be reduced in the New Testament, and certainly would not look for their exclusion from any standing in the church . . . .
>
> (4) Baptism is now by divine authority substituted for circumcision as the initiatory sign and seal of the covenant of grace. Scripture strongly insists on it that circumcision can no more serve in that capacity, ... If baptism did not take its place, the New Testament has no initiatory rite . . . .[6]

Now for a few comments on each of these arguments.

First, Berkhof implies that the national aspect of the Abrahamic Covenant is secondary to the spiritual aspect. This is consistent with Covenant Theology which holds that, (1) God is through with the Hebrews as a nation, and (2) the church has taken up where the Jews left off; any prophetic promise that has not been fulfilled already in the seed of Abraham will be fulfilled in the church. If all this could be proved, Berkhof would have less trouble finding authority for a New Testament ordinance in the Old Testament. But God is not through with the Hebrews as a nation, and the church is not simply a New Testament continuation of this Old Testament people. They are two separate and distinct entities. Once again we see the fallacy of failing to distinguish the dispensational difference between things in the Old Testament and things in the New.

Second, this covenant is still in force so far as Israel is concerned; but it is not and never has been as far as the church is concerned. The national aspect of the Abrahamic Covenant was primarily earthly and included the possession of the land. The destiny of the church is primarily heavenly. Further, circumcision was later made a part of the Mosaic Covenant, and the writer of Hebrews uses much of that book to show the many differences between that covenant and the new covenant. Yet, he never says that any of the ceremonies of the old covenant are to be replaced by baptism.

Third, where is the New Testament Scripture that says the appointment of God by which infants shared in the benefits of the Abrahamic Covenant is carried over into the New Testament? If this were true, certainly the New Testament would have had something definite to say about it. But, remember, the fact that it did not is the reason Pedobaptists must resort to the Old Testament for their authority. The only reason Berkhof gives for the above assumption is that "... we would hardly expect the privileges of such children to be reduced in the New Testament, and certainly would not look for their exclusion from any standing in the Church ...." He said, "Jesus and the apostles did not exclude them, ..." and then gives Scripture that has nothing at all to do with baptism of unbelieving and unregenerate babies.

Fourth, where in the New Testament is baptism by divine authority substituted for circumcision as the initiatory sign and seal of the covenant of grace? The only proof Berkhof gives is that, "If baptism did not take its [circumcision] place, the New Testament has no initiatory rite ...." But Berkhof is adding apples and oranges. Baptism is an initiatory rite for believers; there is no such New Testament rite for infants.

The thrust of these four arguments is that the Abrahamic Covenant is being fulfilled in the church; and therefore, baptism now takes the place of circumcision. Children were circumcised under the old covenant; children should be baptized under the new covenant. But is this true? There are several reasons to believe it is not. Consider, first, the following that is offered by W. D. Nowlin.

> ... To convince you that baptism did not take the place of circumcision, ... *it is sufficient to remind you that Paul was baptized after he was circumcised and that Timothy was circumcised after he was baptized.* If baptism had come in the room and stead of circumcision, then there would have been no place for Paul's baptism, for he had circumcision, and there would have been no place for Timothy's circumcision, for he had baptism (emphasis is his) ....[7]

There is one more reason we shall consider which shows that Old Testament circumcision is not parallel to New Testament baptism. Pedobaptists baptize both male and female babies, but there is no circumcision of female babies in Old Testament practice. This idea came to me sometime ago just before I was to preach on the subject of infant baptism. It was so obvious that I hesitated to mention it for fear it might be thought foolish. Imagine my surprise when, sometime later, I was reading the Appendix to the *Philadelphia Confession of Faith* and came across the following pertaining to circumcision and baptism.

> So it [circumcision] was in the covenant that God made with Abraham and his seed, the sign whereof was appropriated only to the male, notwithstanding that the female seed, as well as the male, were comprehended in the covenant ....

> For that [circumcision] was suited only for the male children; baptism is an ordinance suited for every believer, whether male or

female....[8]

So, if the Pedobaptists could justify their practice of substituting baptism for circumcision it would solve the problem only for male babies. There are other definite differences; but this is enough to show that, under close and logical scrutiny, the parallel between circumcision and baptism breaks down.

VARIOUS OBSERVATIONS

"Baptism is intended for believers and their seed." So say reformed Pedobaptists. Doubtless, many who would not claim the reformed handle would limit infant baptism in this way also. But this is not the case with all baby baptizers. Those who believe that baptism is absolutely essential to salvation think it is their duty to baptize everyone they can get their hands on. Others cite their belief that the covenant promises extend to the thousandth generation (Psalm 105:8-10) as their basis for baptizing almost anyone. However, the relationship of infant baptism to the State-Church idea is possibly the reason (for baptizing all) that has the most far reaching results. In this kind of situation a child has a right to baptism just as he has any other rights by virtue of being a citizen of the state, and he is considered to have a responsibility to be baptized also. In the case of infant baptism this responsibility falls upon the parents. Many have suffered horribly for failing, or rather refusing, to perform this responsibility.

It has already been stated that infant baptism was considered by a number of the Reformers to be necessary if the State-Church was to succeed. Had they followed their stated belief that the Bible was to be followed as their rule of authority for faith and practice, they would have rejected infant baptism. However, to have done so would have meant that they considered many of the civil authorities to be unbaptized; and that would have left them without the political muscle which they considered to be so necessary to the success of their movement. Needless to say, this cooperation on the part of the state was to be used by the Reformers as it had been by the Catholics for the purpose of persecution to coerce others to go their way.

This was not only true in Europe; it made its way to America as well. Notice how it was used by the Puritans in an attempt to gain religious control. Adams writes,

> ... Even the Puritans, who fled from persecution in England, had no idea of religious liberty. They came here to establish their own faith, and to exclude all others; hence they were more rigidly intolerant than the countries whence they had fled from persecution. "Intolerance was a necessary condition of their enterprise. They feared and hated religious liberty" (Here Adams has quoted Dr. Ellis, lecture before the New England Historical Society, March 11, 1860).
>
> All who did not conform to their views, were fined and imprisoned, and whipped and banished; and, as Baptists were especially opposed to religious oppression, the heaviest persecutions fell upon them. Hence, in 1644, a law was passed in Massachusetts against the Baptists, by which it was "ordered and agreed, that if any person or persons within this jurisdiction shall either openly condemn or oppose the baptism of infants, or seduce others to do so, or leave the congregation during the administration of the rite, he shall be sentenced to banishment...."[9]

It can be clearly seen that infant baptism was used as a point upon which to command compliance with an established religion, or one they hoped to establish as the religion of the state. Here it should be noted that their purpose was not to establish Christianity as opposed to paganism, but it was to establish their own particular Christian belief as opposed to all others. What had been used in the old country to accomplish this particular objective was now used in what was to become the United States of America for the same purpose.

There are other ways in which infant baptism is a help to the success of a State-Church; it limits liberty. Some have said that it always produces oppression and persecution wherever it has had the opportunity to develop itself. But how does it further the cause of the State-Church concept? Infant baptism commits a person, while he is still not conscious of it, to a certain church; and, as we have seen, when this child has arrived at years of discretion, he is bound to perform all the duties of church members. He must remain in this church and abide by its regulations and doctrine or turn from that to which he has been committed since infancy. This is a definite limitation of the individual's liberty and goes along with the limitations of liberty that are invariably imposed by a State-Church.

In case you think I am being overly severe in this matter, remember we have seen in previous places that Zwingli turned to the practice of infant baptism as opposed to his first belief. He did this because he was bound to the idea of a State-Church and did not think it could succeed without this Pedobaptist practice.

Perhaps it will be argued that Baptists are guilty of trying to influence their children to be Baptists. Our answer is that any parent who does not try to influence his children to believe and practice the truth as he sees it is derelict in his duty. However, there is a vast difference between the practice of influencing by teaching and admonishing children to believe and do what is right and the practice of doing it for them and then demanding that they not depart from it. No matter how greatly influenced or how well taught a child may be, when he reaches the time when he is responsible, he must make the final choice. A person who holds Baptist principles will defend his right to make this choice.

There is further restraint on a person who is baptized as an infant and then experiences regeneration at a later date. When this happens, parents are almost always unwilling to permit biblical, believers' baptism. The reason they give is that the person has already been baptized; and guilt, in one form or another, is used as a motivational force to prevent him from forsaking the church of his parents, the one in which he was baptized as a tiny infant.

Pedobaptists do not make any provision for a person who was baptized as an infant to be baptized after a genuine experience of salvation. I read this in a book that was written in the last century; and feeling that the information might be out of date, I checked with a Presbyterian pastor. He confirmed that it is still true today. Then it dawned on me; it would have to be true or the Pedobaptists would become Anabaptists. They would be guilty of the same crime for which Catholics and Protestants persecuted the Baptists. Then, if baptism of believers only is the only biblical baptism, Pedobaptist churches prevent one who has been sprinkled as an infant from following the teachings of the Bible in the matter of believers' baptism.

Perhaps this will explain much of why Baptists believe as they do in this matter. May we who bear this name be certain of the biblical basis of our beliefs and having done this, stand for them!

BIBLIOGRAPHY

1. Christian, John T., *A History of the Baptists*. Vol. 1 of 2 vols. Nashville, Tennessee: Broadman Press, 1922, p 199
2. Armitage, Thomas, *History of the Baptists*. New York, New York: Bryan, Taylor & Co., 1890. p 333
3. Ibid.
4. Berkhof, Louis, *Systematic Theology*. Vol. II of 2 vols. Grand Rapids, Michigan: Wm. B. Eerdmans Publishing Co., 1938. p 245
5. Armitage, Ibid., p 334
6. Berkhof, Ibid., pp 241,242
7. Nowlin, William Dudley, D.D., *Fundamentals of the Faith*. Nashville, Tennessee: Sunday School Board of the Southern Baptist Convention, 1926. p 273
8. _____, *The Philadelphia Confession of Faith*. Appendix. Sterling Virginia: Grace Abounding Ministries, n.d. pp 61,62
9. Adams, John Quincy, *Baptists Thorough Reformers*. Rochester, New York: Backus Book Publishers, n.d. p 98

CHAPTER VI
UNHOLY MATRIMONY

In the letters to the seven churches in the book of The Revelation, the third church that is addressed is Pergamos. Many students of the Bible believe the description of these churches gives a preview of the history of the entire church age. If this is true, the church at Pergamos provides an interesting study. The last part of the name of this church is "gamos" and in the Greek language it is the word for marriage. This, together with the chronological location of the message to this church, makes a good case for its representing, prophetically, that part of the church age that began with the "conversion" of the emperor Constantine and the resulting marriage of the church and state.

Constantine placed Christianity on an equal basis with the other religions of the empire and gradually began to favor it. In return, he demanded that the church let him have a good bit to say about its operation. As we have seen in a previous chapter, Constantine became Pontifex Maximus of the church.

Whether Constantine's vision of the cross ever happened is open to question, but there is no question about his part in laying the foundation for the marriage of the state and the church. This was the beginning of the State-Church concept, and it was not long before the coercive power of the state was used to build the church. One church gained the upper hand and became the State-Church, and it had the exclusive right of existence. To it, all must conform. The remainder of church history was colored by this concept, and many died in their quest for freedom to worship God according to the dictates of their conscience rather than submit to the coercion that resulted from this unholy marriage. Soon the doctrine of "two swords" developed, of which we will speak later.

THE POWERS THAT BE

Before continuing, notice that the governmental authorities have seldom been supportive of the true church in this age. Much of the time they have been used in an effort to stamp out the truth. This was first manifest when the Jewish leaders used the power of the Roman Empire to crucify Jesus because it was not lawful for them to put anyone to death (John 18:31). This power of the state was used further in persecution of the apostle Paul and other preachers of the gospel of Jesus Christ. Tradition records the violent deaths of most of the apostles at the hands of the state.

It was at the hands of the Roman Empire that the church suffered its first general persecution. Emperor worship came to prevail in the Roman Empire. At times the Christians were granted toleration under which they would be permitted to worship if they would acknowledge that they were worshipping by permission of the emperor. To them, this amounted to a license from the state; and in effect, it meant that they would be looking to the civil authority, the emperor, as the highest power. Their answer to this was "Jesus is Lord." Rome's answer to them was "death." Christians were thrown to the lions in the Colosseum, used as flaming torches to illuminate the gardens of Nero; and some were sealed in the catacombs, where they had resorted to worship, and left to perish.

The above, however, has nothing to do with the State-Church. It simply shows that governmental powers have often been used against the church and have been hostile to true believers much of the time. The world will always be hostile to the church when its way of life is threatened. It was when the gospel message that Paul preached turned many from idols to serve the living and true God that the Ephesian Silversmith's Local #1 tried to do away with him. Such as this happened many times, but persecution has never been so devastating as when it is done by a union of the state and the church.

THE TABLES ARE TURNED

Almost as soon as the heathen stopped persecuting the church an amazing thing happened; the church started persecuting the heathen and heretics. At times Christians persecuted each other because of difference in doctrine and practice. The persecution was not as severe as it had been and was to become. At this time they did not torture or put people to death, but banishment was common and some died on the way to their place of exile. Many of those who were persecuted as heretics held some of the beliefs that we hold dear today; and as is common in many cases, their beliefs were either blown out of proportion, taken out of context, or they were victims of outright lies.

Although there was much severe persecution brought about by the alliance of the state and the church, there were times when the leaders of the civil government tried to gain the upper hand, and vice versa. One such case involved Henry IV of Germany and Pope Gregory VII. At the center of this struggle was the question of the right of investiture; that is, did the emperor have the authority to appoint men to positions in the Church or did that right belong only to the pope? The outcome was that the emperor was excommunicated and he made a pilgrimage across the Alps in the bitter cold and snow to appear before the pope at Canossa. Here he waited in the courtyard, barefooted and bareheaded in the snow. In the latter part of the afternoon of the third day the door opened and he entered and stood before the pope, Gregory VII. Henry stood before him as a penitent; then he fell to the floor and asked for forgiveness. This was granted and the ban of excommunication was lifted.

But this was not the end. Henry's action had been a clever political ploy. He had actually forced Gregory to grant him absolution, which must be done when one comes as a penitent. The tide turned against Gregory; and in the course of time, Henry marched against Rome and installed the anti-pope of his own choice.[1]

At times the church had the upper hand; at other times the state held sway. However, the most severe persecution occurred when the two worked together. In the Inquisition, those suspected of heresy were called before the Roman Catholic Court. If the accused was found to hold heretical ideas in the eyes of this body, he was required to recant, i.e., deny his heretical beliefs. If he did, he went free; but if he did not, he was handed over to the civil government for punishment because "the Church does not shed blood." Punishment was often death by being burned at the stake. If anyone would not answer the questions of the inquisitors, he was tortured until he either confessed or died at the hands of his tormentors. There were too many of the Waldenses for the Roman Church to deal with in this way, so armies were sent against them and it is said that for twenty years, "blood flowed like water." All over England the Lollards, followers of John Wycliffe, died as martyrs by being burned at the stake. All this was done at the instigation of the Church, but the sentences were executed by governmental powers. To read of these terrible times makes us wonder at the extent of man's inhumanity to man, and this is especially true when the perpetrators claimed to be followers and servants of Jesus.

These conditions still prevailed in the time of the Reformation, and many of the Reformers met fates similar to those of whom we have written. Luther's life was in great danger from the time he nailed his ninety-five theses to the church door in Wittenberg. At one time he was summoned to appear in Rome, and it is quite possible that if he had gone at that time, he would have been burned at the stake as others were during that period. The same could have been true when he appeared before the Diet of Worms. However, circumstances involving the church, the state, and the people worked in such a way that Luther was providentially preserved to continue the work of the Reformation. Eventually, the Reformation prospered so that the power of the papacy was broken to a large extent. Luther was able to bring about religious liberty to a degree. In fact, he even began to teach some of the truths that we hold dear today.

However, the persecuted gradually became the persecutors, and it is said by some historians that the persecution under the Reformers was as severe as it had been under the Roman Church. We have already seen that Zwingli was instrumental in the drowning death of Felix Mantz and others. John Calvin, one of the greatest of the Reformers and a man who is considered by many to be one of the greatest biblical scholars of all time, was instrumental in the death of Servetus, who was burned at the stake on October 27, 1553. Servetus had been tried and convicted of heresy, and he was guilty of holding some strange ideas. But how strange that one who knew the Scriptures, as Calvin is said to have known them, would be so intimately involved in such an act.

And involved he was. His followers have tried to excuse his action in this matter by saying that it was either Servetus or Calvin; or that this was just a product of the times, that burning heretics was in vogue at that point in history. Some said that Calvin tried to avert such a severe penalty and to have the sentence commuted to some form of death rather than death by burning; but if this is true, it was because Calvin wanted him to be executed as a civil offender. Death by fire was reserved for those who were guilty of religious offenses.[2] The fact is, Calvin believed in death for heretics, and he was applauded by other Reformers. The Reformer, Melanchthon, wrote, "The Church owes and always will owe a debt of gratitude to you for having put the heretic to death." He and a group of his defenders produced a defense of his actions which was published in 1554, a short time after Servetus perished.[3] Christian shows Calvin's feeling in these matters by quoting him concerning the Anabaptists. He said that ". . . Anabaptists and reactionists should alike be put to death." He said further, ". . . These altogether deserve to be well punished by the sword, seeing that they do conspire against God, ..."[4]

The State-Church concept has produced persecution from time to time since its inception. Sometimes the ones to be the recipients of persecution depended on the one who had the greatest pull with those in power in the civil government. If the Catholics prevailed, the Reformers were persecuted as well as the Anabaptists; if the Reformers prevailed, the Anabaptists caught it. At times, persecution ceased for a period but then returned.

RHYME AND REASON

Certainly, those claiming to be Christians could not have been so cruel in persecuting others to the death, and such a horrendous death at that, without reasons for doing it and without some purpose in doing so. They claimed both. Let us look at the purpose first and then at the reasons.

The avowed purpose of coercion was to be rid of heretics, if they could not force them to believe and be good members of the church. However, the charge of heresy was sometimes based on false accusations. For instance, at times the charge against the "heretics" was that they were against any civil rule. This was not true. It is true that they allowed no civil rule in spiritual matters; but for the most part, that was as far as it went. Many attest to the fact that they were among the most law abiding citizens of the land. They just believed in freedom of conscience or soul liberty in their relationship to God. This charge was, no doubt, used as a coverup for the real reasons, which ranged from their refusing to have their children baptized to their refraining from attending Mass because they considered the doctrine of Transubstantiation as sacrificing Jesus over and over again. These "heretics" believed that He offered one sacrifice for sins forever, and they believed civil authorities had no jurisdiction in these things. However, civil control of spiritual matters was necessary to retain and maintain the State-Church.

Further, their purpose was full of fallacy, especially as related to the Reformers, because their belief was inconsistent with the practice. Here was a body of people who believed strongly in the sovereignty of

God, which included a belief that none could come to God unless drawn of the Holy Spirit, i.e., unless he were one of the elect. But, in practice, they tried to coerce elect and non-elect alike to believe. This is the height of inconsistency.

Now, what about reasons that could make the union of church and state and the resultant coercion on their part right in their eyes? First, consider the teaching of Augustine concerning the millennium. Remember, we have already seen the great influence of Augustine on the dogma of the Catholic Church. Augustine taught that the millennium was a period of time between the incarnation of Christ and His second advent, and it was during this time that the church would conquer the world. Cairns says that it was this teaching that led to the Roman emphasis upon the Church of Rome as the universal church destined to bring all within its fold.[5] Thus, the Church of God becomes the same as the Kingdom of God on earth. In a kingdom there must be rule, control. There is no room for anyone, outside of this realm, with opposing beliefs. So coercion was employed, judicially, by the church but with the state as its instrument of execution. The purpose was to bring all within the realm of this church and build the kingdom, a kingdom with its head in Rome, but with its tentacles reaching to the uttermost part of the earth. But these tentacles choked instead of converting.

However, even with the erroneous teaching of Augustine concerning the millennium, the idea of a *functioning*, universal church on earth cannot be found in the New Testament. It is quite evident that this idea was brought about as a result of a misunderstanding of the word "church."

"Ecclesia," the Greek word from which we get our word "church," was already in use before Jesus used it of His church. It meant a local assembly of people who were called out of their homes or businesses and assembled to attend to public affairs. Prescribed conditions of membership are implied. This assembly was an independent body; and it was autonomous, i.e., selfgoverning. This Greek word is used 117 times in the New Testament; at least 92 times it is used in its primary sense of called-out ones assembled. The other times it is used do not take away from this primary meaning. A New Testament church, then, is a local assembly of called-out, baptized believers who hold the New Testament as their only law. Therefore, according to the New Testament, the Catholic idea of themselves as a universal (universal means Catholic) church is wrong.

All true Christians are in the body of Christ, but they are not assembled. When Jesus comes again, all these will assemble; and at that time they will be a functioning church. Further, it will be a local church, not a universal church.

Perhaps it will help in understanding this if we think of a church as a building, as the New Testament presents it. All of the material for it might be delivered to the building site. All that the building will ever consist of is there, but it is not a building until it is assembled. In the strictest sense of interpretation, a church does not exist during the week. Its members are scattered throughout the community. It becomes a church when it is assembled, on Sunday or whenever. Bible translators could have properly used the word "assembly" instead of "church." If they had done so, perhaps there would have been less confusion about a universal church functioning on earth.

Now, what about the Reformers? It is interesting that reformed churches to this day have believed, substantially, in the millennial teaching of Augustine; and evidently, many of them have missed the meaning of the church. This millennial belief is also evident among many who call themselves Reformed Baptists. This would indicate that there remained in the Reformers then, and in reformed churches now, something of the universal church idea; and that they have not been willing to separate themselves completely from the Roman Church, especially from the idea that they are the church, and all who are outside are not part of the true church.

That a complete departure from the Roman Church has not been made by them is indicated by the following statements taken from "Letters to the Editor," U. S. News and World Report of December 5, 1983. I quote, "Anglicanism does not think of itself as founded by Henry VIII or even Elizabeth I . . . . We think of the Church of England as the Catholic Church in England, separated from Roman jurisdiction when Elizabeth I became Queen in 1558." Further, a Lutheran pastor wrote, "Actually, it is Rome for whom we are prayerfully waiting to seek reconciliation and union with us." While these statements are open to some interpretation, they do show that there never has been a complete departure. There is no doubt that Augustinian millennialism has had a definite effect on the Catholic Church, the Reformers, and on reformed churches today; and that this teaching helped lay the foundation for State-Church coercion.

But there is more. These of whom we have just spoken would certainly be expected to seek biblical reason for taking such extreme measures. We would especially expect this of the Reformers. And where did they find such reasons? In the New Testament, they claimed! First, in Luke 22:38, the disciples said, ". . . Lord, behold, here are two swords . . . ." From this the church built the doctrine that they had two swords with which to do their kingdom work. One was the sword of the Spirit to be used by the church, i.e., the preaching of the Word. If that failed, they had the sword of steel to be used for the church by the civil authorities, the state, for physical coercion. Of course, they overlooked the fact that Jesus rebuked Peter for using one of the swords in a physical fashion. But they overlooked a number of other things as well.

Other Scripture was used. Again they resorted to Augustine who taught that the words of Jesus, ". . . Go out into the highways and hedges, and compel them to come in, . . ." (Luke 14:23) meant that coercion was to be used to build a church.

Beza provided a proof text, if such it can be called. Verduin quotes his reasoning from two well known passages in the book of Acts. Beza wrote,

". . . With what power, pray, did Peter put to death Ananias and

> Sapphira? And with what power did Paul smite Elymas blind? Was it with the power that is vested in the Church? Of course not. Well then, it must have been with the power that is vested in the magistrate, there being no third kind of power .... [6]

It is not even necessary to say that such reasoning is the result of faulty interpretation, and more probably, of outright dishonest dealing with what he knew these Scriptures to mean.

No doubt, there were more arguments put forth in an attempt to justify this immoral and unbiblical practice; but these are sufficient to show that they provided no sound foundation for it.

THERE OUGHT TO BE A LAW

Perhaps all of us, at one time or another, have thought there ought to be a law against at least some of the outlandish religious cults that exist in this day. For instance, the cult led by Jim Jones and its freakish philosophy of religion that led to the Jonestown massacre in which nearly one thousand people perished. The Moonies would be likely candidates if we were making a list of those we have thought should be outlawed. There are others who work within our local communities, peddling their pernicious propaganda and clearly deceiving the people by their false doctrine. There is no doubt, cults abound that are leading young people and adults away from God, their families, and friends and into the night of spiritual darkness.

Why not outlaw such people as this? Well, our forebears evidently never thought of that. At different times they, no doubt, thought of laws that would make it a crime to persecute others that held beliefs that differed from theirs. And, no doubt, they opposed these opposing beliefs with all that was within them; but they believed that everyone had a right to hold their beliefs, no matter how far out they might be. Furthermore, they were willing to defend this right of others; and they demanded this right for themselves.

Through all of the State-Church development and the resultant persecution there developed or, perhaps, came to light, the Baptist distinctive of separation of church and state and freedom of conscience, or soul liberty. This meant, simply, that the government did not have the right to establish any one church as the State-Church and demand that everyone belong to it. It meant that everyone has the freedom to worship God according to the dictates of his own conscience without interference or coercion from any outside human source, especially from the state. It does not mean, as some seem to believe today, that anyone in the government cannot also be active in a church, or that anyone in the church cannot have a definite voice in the affairs of state. It simply means that the state cannot dictate to anyone in spiritual matters. We will see more about this in the following chapter as we study this question as it is related to our own country.

There are several passages of Scripture that have a bearing on this matter. First, we shall consider two of them that, at first glance, seem to be contradictory. In his letter to the saints in Rome, Paul wrote,

> Let every soul be subject unto the higher powers. For there is no power but of God: the powers that be are ordained of God. Whosoever therefore resisteth the power, resisteth the ordinance of God: and they that resist shall receive to themselves damnation (Romans 13:1,2).

But how did this square with the practice of the apostles in their direct confrontation with the authorities? Consider the account of the actions of Peter and others when they were arrested and asked to give an answer for their action in preaching the gospel.

> And when they had brought them, they set them before the council: and the high priest asked them, Saying, Did not we straitly command you that ye should not teach in this name? and, behold, ye

have filled Jerusalem with your doctrine, and intend to bring this man's blood upon us. Then Peter and the other apostles answered and said, We ought to obey God rather than men (Acts 5:27-29).

Notice, a seeming contradiction is not necessarily an actual contradiction. There is no contradiction between the instructions given by Paul and the action of the apostles that is related above. In the first, Paul is speaking of civil powers; but Peter and the others stood before religious authorities. Notice, however, that the religious authorities evidently sent civil officers to arrest, imprison, and deliver the Christians to them, showing a union of religious and civil powers intruding into spiritual matters. In such matters, the accused claimed that they were not bound to obey man, but they were bound to obey God. This is a clear declaration of the Baptist distinctive that calls for freedom of conscience and the resultant belief that the state has no authority in spiritual matters. This freedom is absolute if the church or state acts independently or if they act together. Christians are to bow before the state in the matter of secular things but not in that which is spiritual.

Another passage of Scripture gives the proper balance that we, as Christians, should seek to maintain. It is a principle laid down by none other than Jesus. This principle was given in answer to a question that the Pharisees and Herodians had asked. We shall consider just the question and the answer.

> ... Tell us therefore, What thinkest thou? Is it lawful to give tribute to Caesar, or not? .... Then saith he unto them, Render therefore unto Caesar the things which are Caesar's; and unto God the things that are God's (Matthew 22:17,21).

This clearly shows that the church and the state are not to be one and the same; neither are they to be opposing forces. Both are ordained of God, both being ministers of God and having their proper functions, but each in its own realm. The church is responsible in spiritual matters; the state is responsible in civil matters. This is the teaching of Scripture, and it leaves each individual free to determine what he will believe without being forced to act against his conscience.

In closing, it must be noted that our freedom to worship God according to the dictates of our conscience is a freedom only as far as our relationship to human government is concerned. No such right exists pertaining to our relationship to God. The conscience of man is defiled by the fall and is not an accurate guide in spiritual matters. God demands that we worship Him according to the instructions given in His Word, the Bible. Our freedom is that which gives us liberty to interpret this Word without outside interference from man and to worship God accordingly.

Man has freedom from worship as far as man's authority is concerned, but no such freedom exists as far as God's authority is concerned. God demands worship from his creature, man; and He requires that that worship be according to His Word.

BIBLIOGRAPHY

1. Kuiper, B. K., *The Church in History*. Grand Rapids, Michigan: Wm. B. Eerdmans Publishing Co., 1951. Summary
2. Verduin, Leonard, *The Reformers and Their Stepchildren*. Grand Rapids, Michigan: Baker Book House, 1964. p 52
3. Ibid., p 53
4. Christian, John T., *A History of the Baptists*. Vol. I of 2 vols. Nashville Tennessee: Broadman Press, 1926, pp 198,199
5. Cairns, Earle E., *Christianity Through the Centuries*. Grand Rapids, Michigan: Zondervan Publishing House, 1954, 1967. p 161
6. Verduin, Ibid., p 54

CHAPTER VII
SWEET LAND OF LIBERTY

Familiar phrases remind us of our heritage of freedom, phrases like "land of the free" and "let freedom ring." My grandfather used to begin his prayers by thanking God that we could assemble peacefully and "worship God according to the dictates of our conscience and none dare molest or make us afraid." I often wondered if he realized the full import of that freedom for which he thanked his heavenly Father. Perhaps few living today, in these United States, have any idea of what our freedom frees us from. You who have read thus far know something of the awful things that have been suffered by those who worshipped God as they believed they should, according to His Word; but we have only been able to give a few examples of their suffering. The magnitude and extent of this suffering staggers the imagination. Further, it is impossible to enter into their feelings because there is no way for us to feel as they felt by just reading about their experiences. To say that it was horrible beyond imagination is a gross understatement.

During the lifetime of those born in this country, we have known freedom such as the rest of the world has seldom known. Consequently, we are prone to believe that it always has been like this, that it is like this throughout the world, and that it always will be. But it has not always been like this, even in this sweet land of liberty. It is true that many fled the old world to escape religious persecution; it is also true that many of them came to establish a State-Church that would favor them and over which they would have authority. And, although they had been persecuted because of their religious beliefs, they now became the persecutors of those who did not believe their way and do the way they wanted them to do. Religious intoleration was rampant in the colonies, and freedom was slow in coming. It finally came about because of the efforts of many outside the established church who were willing to fight, to the death if necessary, against the "powers that be" having any control over the church.

The beliefs and attitudes of those who came to the New World to escape religious persecution are interesting. The Puritans believed that a union of the church and state was a political necessity. They also wanted religious liberty for themselves and perfect toleration, but they were not willing for others to have it. They wanted their church to be the established church of the land. Armitage said, "A facetious writer may be allowed to say that the Puritans came to this country 'to worship God according to their own conscience, and to prevent other people from worshipping him according to theirn,' ...."[1]

In the early part of the seventeenth century, sermons were preached against religious toleration. Consider the following examples. The first condemned anyone who was willing

> ... to tolerate any religion or discrepant way of religion, besides his own, or is not sincere in it. There is no truth but one, and of the persecution of true religion and toleration of false, the last is far the worst. It is said that men ought to have liberty of conscience, and that it is persecution to debar them from it. I can rather stand amazed than reply to this. It is an astonishment that the brains of men should be parboiled in such impious ignorance.[2]

And another said of the outcry of some for liberty of conscience,

> ... This is the great Diana of the libertines of this age. I look upon toleration as the first born of all iniquities. If it should be brought forth amongst us, you may call it Gad, a troop cometh, a troop of all manner of abominations....[3]

At this early time, most of the Puritans thought it was impossible for people of different sects to live together, peaceably, in the same settlements. Even when they were the recipients of persecution, they still stood against toleration.

Concerning the Presbyterians of this time, Christian quotes Ruffini.

> ... So resolutely and blindly did the Presbyterians profess the principles of the rigid Calvinism, that they became absolutely irreconcilable with any other religious denomination and as belligerent as the most implacable Catholic. Their supreme ideal was the realization of the kingdom of Christ on earth .... Indeed, one of them said, "If the devil were given the choice of re-establishing in the kingdom the episcopal [intolerance] or granting toleration, he [the devil] would certainly declare in favor of the latter." And another added, "I would rather find myself buried in the grave than live to see this intolerable toleration."[4]

The Congregationalists established their government as a theocracy. But they patterned it after the Jewish form of government in the Old Testament. This meant a union of church and state since, in the Old Testament, the state and the people of God were one and the same. Accordingly, under this form of government, no one was permitted to hold office or even to enjoy his full civil rights unless he was a member of the established (state) church. This will play an important part later in this chapter as we consider the drama surrounding the passing of the First Amendment to the Constitution.

In early colonial times, most Baptists did not seem to be in churches of their own but were forced to attend churches with which they were not in doctrinal agreement. They had ways of showing their disapproval of such practices as that of infant baptism, etc. They would stand with their backs turned to the minister as he was performing the ceremony, or they would walk out of the assembly in such a way as to show that they did not approve of the ordinance being administered in this way. One of them showed disrespect by sleeping in church and was arrested, tried, and punished for such things as, ". . . 'for common sleeping at the public exercise upon the Lord's day, and for striking him that waked him,' and was 'severely whipped' for the same...."[5] When John Clarke was forced to attend the State-Church, it is said, "...When he was taken in he removed his hat and 'civilly saluted them,' but when he had been conducted to a seat he put on his hat, 'opened my book and fell to reading'...."[6] More about this brother later.

It must be remembered that these colonists had recently come or were descended from those who had come from Europe, many of them from England where such government was the norm and punishment for religious infractions was common. We would expect this kind of thing to continue in the New World, and continue it did. It was during this period of time that the Salem witch hunt and subsequent hanging of twenty who were accused of being witches happened. This was done with the approval and possibly at the instigation of Cotton Mather, son of Increase Mather and pastor of the North Church (Congregational). So we need not be surprised to learn that most sects believed in a State-Church and in severe punishment for those who did not conform. Apparently, the only two exceptions were the Baptists and Quakers, and these were two of the most persecuted peoples in the New World.

Perhaps a knowledge of the things that were suffered by Christians in the early days of our own country will help us to be more appreciative of the freedoms we now enjoy. One of the hardships which was caused by the State-Church union was that the ministers of churches outside of the established church were not considered legitimate. Therefore, marriages performed by them were not legal, and the children of such unions were considered illegitimate. Another hardship was caused by the people being taxed to support the established church. This was burdensome, even when the dissenters were allowed to attend their own church, since there was little financial means left for its support.

However, these things pale into significance when we consider the cruel and unusual punishment that was employed against any who opposed the State-Church, especially the Baptists and Quakers. Consider

A PEOPLE FOR HIS NAME

a few examples.

Thomas Painter had become a Baptist. His wife was a member of the established church, and he would not allow her to have their infant child baptized. He was brought before the authorities and ordered to "cease and desist." When he did not, he was again brought before them and ordered to be whipped.

Laws against the Quakers were enacted, laws which became increasingly severe for repeated transgressions. Later they were ordered to be arrested and if found guilty, to be banished on pain of death. Christian describes the execution of this sentence.

> . . . In carrying out the sentence of banishment, even women, stripped to the waist, and tied to a cart's tail, were whipped from town to town, and carried on a two days' journey into the wilderness, among wolves and bears. To cap the climax of intolerance, Quakers were hanged in 1659, 1660, and 1661 . . . .[7]

Backus tells of the execution of several Quakers by hanging.

> On October 20th, Robinson, Stevenson and Mary Dyre, received the sentence of death. It was executed upon the two men, the 27th. The woman was brought with them to the gallows, but at the intercession of her son of Newport and others, she was then reprieved and sent away. Returning again the next spring, she was hanged, June 1st, 1660 . . . .[8]

In fairness to the rulers who were responsible for these atrocities it should be said that these were banished on pain of death for religious reasons. However, the two men refused to depart, their reason being that they wanted to "try your bloody law unto death." This made them guilty of civil disobedience, and for that they were put to death.

Mary Dyre was not reprieved at the gallows as the language of Backus seems to indicate. This was done before the magistrates several days earlier on condition that she leave the area. But she was required to stand on the gallows with a rope around her neck while the other two were executed. Her return after the sentence of banishment made her guilty of civil disobedience also, and for this she was hanged. This makes these cases different from that of many of the Baptists who were punished severely because they insisted on worshipping God according to their understanding of the Scriptures.

One account of the persecution of Baptists in Massachusetts tells of the merciless whipping of Obadiah Holmes. He, together with pastor John Clarke and another brother, James Crandall, had gone to the home of an old Christian brother, William Whitter, who lived in the town of Lyn (or Lin). On Sunday, they decided to hold services in his home. However, Whitter had been in trouble with the authorities several times before, and it is possible that this might have precipitated the events that transpired that day.

Whatever the cause, while these men were holding private worship services in his home, Clarke, Crandall, and Holmes were arrested and the following day were taken to Boston where "without producing accuser, witness, jury, or any law," they were fined various amounts or they were to be "well whipped." Friends paid the fines of Clarke and Crandall and would have paid that of Obadiah Holmes, but he would not allow it. He felt that to have done so would have been an admission of wrong doing.

On September 6, 1651, Holmes was stripped at the whipping-post and received thirty lashes with a corded whip. Although he was beaten until his flesh quivered and blood streamed from his body, he said to the magistrates, "You have struck me as with roses." Nevertheless, he was not able to rest except on his knees and elbows for some days and perhaps weeks afterwards. According to Armitage, the crime for which he was so severely punished was "hearing a sermon in a private manner."

The conditions of which we have just written existed in the Massachusetts colony, but the other colonies had similar laws. In most of them religious toleration was unknown. To avoid being unduly laborious, we will only look at conditions in the Virginia colony.

The charter of Virginia made the Church of England the established church. Whipping and servitude were some of the penalties for breaking the laws of the church. Speaking against the Trinity or the Christian religion was punishable by death. In some places branding and cutting off ears were other forms of punishment. The use of the stocks seems to have been common, and imprisonment and banishment were frequent. Imprisonment was in jails where fleas abounded and lack of sanitary conditions made life intolerable. Some have suggested that these laws were too cruel to be rigidly enforced but there is much evidence that they were. Testimony can be given to show that this period was one of great suffering on the part of those who were willing to bow before God but not before the state.

The suffering because of religious intolerance during the colonial period is looked upon by Christian as

> ... almost incredible. That men should be whipped, imprisoned, banished, ears cut off, tongue bored with a hot iron and put to death in a barbarous manner; that women should be tied to the tail end of a cart, dragged from town to town and whipped along the way, stripped to the waist, and finally carried into the wilderness and left among wolves and bears to die, all for some religious belief, now held by most men to be harmless, all happening in this country in the last three hundred years, requires the fullest confirmation. Yet the facts are not disputed.[9]

All this happened in what was to become the land of the free, a land where we have enjoyed religious liberty, freedom of conscience, and soul liberty all of our lives. And, it was through the efforts of many of these who had been persecuted or who knew of this persecution that we enjoy our freedom today. Many of those who were champions in the fight for freedom were, understandably, Baptists.

FAITH OF OUR FATHERS

Gradually, the intolerant became more tolerant; not willingly, but circumstances conspired to force a degree of toleration in the colonies. Still, this degree of toleration did not give complete religious freedom that the Baptists desired. There was still a price to pay for holding Christian beliefs and practices that differed from those of the established church. It was not until the colonists began to chafe under the unjust laws imposed upon them by George III, King of England, and the unfair practices of taxation without representation that these conditions began to change by a more satisfactory and permanent solution. As the colonists fought the Revolutionary War for their independence from England and began to draft the Constitution that was to be the basis for their self-government, the Baptists and others were fighting a battle of their own, a battle for religious independence from the State-Church. In places where Baptists were strongest, their love of liberty has been credited with inspiring many to join in fighting for their civil independence. Many Baptists fought in this war; but when it was over, they found that there was still to be fighting if they were to enjoy true religious independence and liberty. In this battle they proved themselves both willing and able; but as they were to discover, much time would pass before they realized their goal.

Jefferson said that by the time of the Revolution, two-thirds of the population of Virginia had become Dissenters. They were, for the most part, Baptists, Quakers, and by this time, Presbyterians. Jefferson had been in close contact with the Baptist church of Buck Mountain in Albemarle, Monticello. It is believed that the impression made on him greatly influenced him as he wrote the first draft of the Declaration of Independence. Copies of his correspondence with this church are available today.

After the war, much time passed as the framers of the Constitution hammered out this document. Finally, it was adopted by the Constitutional Convention and submitted to the states for ratification on September 17, 1787. Ratification by nine of the thirteen states was necessary. Immediately, it met with opposition from all of them for various reasons. The one with which we shall concern ourselves is that it was felt that it did not provide sufficient guarantees of religious freedom. The only mention of the subject of religion was in Article VI which stated, "No religious test shall ever be required, as a qualification to any office or public trust under the United States."

The records of the Colonial Convention, June 20, 1776, reveals that a group of Baptists in Prince William County had sent a petition to this convention in which they asked

> ... that they be allowed to worship God in their own way, without interruption; that they be permitted to maintain their own ministers and none others; that they may be married, buried and the like without paying the clergy of other denominations; that, *these things granted*, they will gladly unite with their brethren, and to the utmost of their ability promote the common cause[10] (Emphasis is Armitage's).

It is quite evident that these were the sentiments of other Baptists as well.

However, when the war was over, victory was won, and independence from England had been purchased at a great price, there were still no guarantees of religious liberty or evidence that the petition of the Baptists had been looked upon with favor. Dissatisfaction with the scant provision for religious liberty that the Constitution contained was manifest by Baptists in all of the states. However, Virginia became their great battlefield. Many political and social leaders, as well as religious leaders, were opposed to the Constitution. Armitage says Patrick Henry opposed the ratification of this document by Virginia because he believed it "squinted toward monarchy and gave no guarantee of religious liberty." But the Constitution was ratified, even though

Henry had submitted a number of amendments, demanding that they be engrafted before Virginia would approve it. Madison agreed that amendments were needed but believed delay in ratification would bring the danger of disunity and so urged its ratification, which was done by Virginia on June 26, 1788. In addition, it was recommended by the Convention that these amendments be embodied in the Constitution. This would alter the Federal Constitution in such a way as to include religious liberty in the fundamental law of the land.

Immediately, Baptists went to work. Elder John Leland was sent to the Baptists of other states to secure their cooperation. Baptist worthies such as Drs. James Manning, Samuel Stillman, and Isaac Backus had worked in Massachusetts to secure ratification. Now, Baptists organized to influence those in high places. They consulted with Madison and wrote to President Washington. Their letter was written by Elder Leland and delivered by a special delegation. It received a favorable response. What an outcry this would elicit today from those who think that any Christian voice concerning matters of state is a violation of the First Amendment.

No Baptist would claim that they were solely responsible for the passage of the amendments that are now known as the Bill of Rights; but there is no doubt that their influence was great, and it is felt by some that they held a balance of power in this matter. In the end, Madison brought a number of Constitutional Amendments before the House of Representatives. Among them was Article I, which was to become the hallowed First Amendment.

> Congress shall make no law respecting an establishment of religion, or prohibiting the free exercise thereof, or abridging the freedom of speech or of the press, or prohibiting the free exercise thereof, or the right of the people peaceably to assemble and to petition the government for a redress of grievances.

Of this Amendment, Armitage commented,

A PEOPLE FOR HIS NAME

> ... Thus, the contemned, spurned and hated old Baptist doctrine of soul-liberty, for which blood had been shed for centuries, was not only engrafted into the organic law of the United States, but for the first time in the formation of a great nation it was made its chief corner-stone....[11]

This amendment did not immediately do away with state churches; for, at the time of the First Amendment's passage, over one-third of the colonies had established churches. In some of the states, dissenting churches were still taxed, and they still endured some oppression at the hands of the established church. But the foundation had been laid that was to develop into the religious freedom that we enjoy today.

STORM CLOUDS

It would be a sad mistake on our part to believe that our religious liberty is permanent. There have been times in the past when Christians have enjoyed religious freedom to an extent. When a certain ruler was on the throne, they were allowed to worship without suffering persecution; however, when another came into power, persecution came again. Persecution, not liberty, seems to have been the norm throughout much of the past; and there are ominous signs today that our liberties that we have thought were guaranteed by the First Amendment are in grave danger. There is evidence that these guarantees have been greatly weakened by decisions of the Supreme Court, decisions that were based on what this amendment has come to mean in the light of past decisions, tradition, and public opinion instead of viewing it in the light of history and the intent of those who framed it.

It should be well understood that, contrary to the beliefs of many, the First Amendment and the doctrine of separation of church and state were never intended to keep Christians from having a voice in the affairs of state. The intent was to keep the powers of government from meddling in the affairs of the church or in the spiritual affairs of individuals. However, several recent cases show that our courts now believe they have the right of control in the spiritual realm. Consider the following cases closely and carefully, for they have far reaching implications.

THE CASE OF ROBIN POLIN

In April 1983, eighteen year old Robin Polin, who was deaf and mute, became a Christian and abandoned the faith of her family. This might not have caused a great problem except for the fact her family was Jewish. As might be expected under such circumstances, her father told her that unless she conformed to his religious views she would not be welcome in his home. Rather than give up her newfound faith, she left. Immediately her parents went to court in an attempt to have her declared incompetent. After a trial which lasted five days, Special District Judge Robert Frank ruled that she was "judgmentally immature." According to the laws of the state, she was regarded as incompetent. Because of this, she was placed in the custody of an older sister.

Late in 1983 the Oklahoma Supreme Court, in an 8 to 1 decision, overturned the decision of the lower court. Concerning this decision, Christianity Today reported,

> ... The state's highest court ruled that Polin's rights guaranteeing the free exercise of religion had been violated. The court labeled the issue of her judgmental immaturity "camouflage," and described Polin's beliefs as "consistent and specific ideals which have motivated her to desire a career as a Christian minister to the deaf."[12]

The decision of the Supreme Court is, of course, good news to those who love liberty; but the fact that a lower court showed a lack of understanding of the foundation of religious liberty and intruded into this matter of conscience shows a threat to religious freedom. It is, at best, a serious violation of the principle of separation of church and state.

THE CASE OF MARIAN GUINN

Marian Guinn was a member of a small rural church in Oklahoma. She was having an affair with a local man; her affair was a well known fact. Ms. Guinn was confronted privately several times by the church elders and counseled to repent or the church would withdraw fellowship from her. She refused to repent; they withdrew fellowship.

Notice, churches are instructed by Scripture to withdraw from, or expel, members who are guilty of sexual sin. In writing to Timothy, Paul said that the rebuke was to be public so others also may fear (I Timothy 5:20).

Regardless of this, Ms. Guinn did not take kindly to this action. She hired an attorney and sued the church for more than a million dollars. She charged invasion of privacy in spite of the fact that her affair was well known. The court rejected motions to dismiss which, in my opinion, should have been granted on the grounds that it had no jurisdiction in this case. It also ruled in favor of Ms. Guinn and awarded her $400,000. The verdict will, no doubt, be appealed and it is hoped, will be reversed. If it is not, it will mean that the state can hold churches liable for enforcing biblical standards on its members. It will also constitute an outrageous invasion by the state into the business of the church. It could mean that no biblical standards could be required for membership, and this would cut the heart from the distinctive that Baptists hold dear. Further, it could well lead to the destruction of all the religious liberties that have been purchased at so great a cost by our forebears.

THE STATE VERSUS THE CHURCH

Faith Baptist Church of Louisville, Nebraska, has been in trouble with the state for a number of years because they do not have teachers in their school that are certified by the State and are graduates of State-approved schools. The church feels that the background in secular humanism that such teachers would have disqualifies them from teaching in private schools that have a conservative Christian perspective. To be certified, their school would also have to have a State-approved curriculum of secular humanism. To be thus certified would destroy the very reason for the existence of their school.

The question is not one of quality education, since their students have scored from one to three years above the average in Nebraska. Pastor and parents are willing to have their children submit each year to standardized tests to insure that they are educated to read, write, compute, and understand their country's history and form of government, as required by the State.

In spite of this, the state padlocked the church; threw the pastor in jail where he stayed for four months, bodily removed eighty-five ministers from the sanctuary, and sent seven fathers to jail and issued bench warrants for the arrests of their wives.

A Nebraska Senator has been quoted as saying,

> We have to control church schools because fundamental, bible-believing Christians do not have the right to indoctrinate their children in their faith, because we, the State, are preparing ALL children for the year 2000 when America will be part of the one world global society and their children won't fit in.

Consider further,

> . . . Several Amish families from Nebraska, rather than com-

promise their convictions, left the State and "some did so only after their possessions were sold at public auction by the sheriff to pay for fines they could not pay or would not pay because of what they considered unconstitutional levies."[13]

These accounts will repulse some, even professed believers, not against the state, but against those who are trying to stand for religious liberty. We would do well to remember that we would not have enjoyed this liberty throughout most of our lives if it had not been for Christians, many of them prominent pastors, who were willing to hazard themselves in their fight for constitutional guarantees of religious liberty. If we do not have men of like mind and caliber today, our religious freedom will be a thing of the past. What a sorry heritage for our children and grandchildren.

It is said that when that indomitable soldier acclaimed by many to be the greatest military genius ever born on this side of the Atlantic, Stonewall Jackson, lay dead because of wounds received on the battlefield at Chancellorsville, one of his devoted officers, bending low over the lifeless corpse, touched the cold hand and said, "If you meet with Caesar tonight, tell him we still make war." Today, we need Christians who will say to their Commander-in-Chief, "If you meet with our Baptist fathers who stood and fought and suffered and died for the right to worship God and believe and practice His Word according to the dictates of their conscience without interference from state or church, tell them we still make war!" And as we fight may we continue to pray,

Our fathers' God, to Thee, Author of liberty,
To Thee we sing:
Long may our land be bright with freedom's Holy Light;
Protect us by thy might, Great God, Our King.

BIBLIOGRAPHY

1. Armitage, Thomas, *History of the Baptists*. New York, New York: Bryan, Taylor & Co., 1890. p 624
2. Christian, John T., *A History of the Baptists*. Vol. II of 2 vols. Nashville, Tennessee: Broadman Press, 1926. p 20
3. Ibid., p 20
4. Ibid., pp 20,21
5. Armitage, Ibid., p 687
6. Ibid., p 687
7. Christian, Ibid. p 60
8. Backus, Isaac, *A History of New England...Baptists*. Vol. I of 3 vols. Newton, Massachusetts: Backus Historical Society, 1871. pp 262,263
9. Christian, Ibid., pp 61,62
10. Armitage, Ibid., p 798
11. Ibid., p 807
12. _____, *"Can a Deaf Mute Jew Become a Christian? A Court Says Yes."* Christianity Today, February 3, 1984. p 46
13. Buffington, J. B., *"Government Wants Control Over Christian Schools."* The Lakeland Ledger, February 11, 1984. n.p.

CHAPTER VIII
THE PROBLEM OF THE PENDULUM

The pendulum of a properly working clock swings first one way and then the other, always to the extreme. If it stopped short of this, it would not cause the clock to keep time accurately; but if it stopped in the middle, the clock would be dead. Man also has a tendency to go from one extreme to the other; but when he does, he often finds himself in a pit of problems. When he seeks solutions to these problems by walking in the middle of the road, he finds himself so compromised that his power is gone because of lack of conviction. Such a situation confronts us in this chapter as we consider the Baptist distinctive of an equal brotherhood of believers and compare it to what actually happened during much of the history of the church. We will not find the solution in going to either extreme to which the church has gone at one time or another; nor will we find it in the middle of the road. The solution will be found in the practice of the balanced teachings of the Bible.

We noticed, in a previous chapter, that the messages to the seven churches in the book of The Revelation are thought by some Bible scholars to be prophetic of the entire church age. If this is true, the message to the Ephesian Church indicates that a problem was already showing itself at an early time, possibly at the end of the apostolic age or very soon thereafter. This problem is manifest in the mention of the hatred the Ephesian Church had for the deeds of the Nicolaitans, which deeds Jesus also hated. A little later, in the message to the church of Pergamos, we learn that what had been "deeds" at Ephesus had become "doctrine" there. But what was the error of the Nicolaitans?

Out of several suggestions, the one that seems most plausible comes from a meaning that is derived from two Greek words that make up the word, *Nicolaitans*. One of them is nikao, from nikan, "to conquer." The other is laos which means, "the people," or "laity." The meaning would be "to conquer the people." The error is that of dividing the church of God into an unequal brotherhood composed of the "clergy" and the "laity" with the clergy ruling over the laity. It is the practice of priestly assumption of authority over the people, of their claim that they had access to God that the people did not have, and of their requiring the people to come to them in order to get in touch with God. Some of its results were the doctrine of the necessity of confession of sins to the priests, priestly absolution, i.e., priests forgiving confessors of their sins, and transubstantiation, in which a priest was necessary to turn the bread and wine into the body and blood of Jesus before it would be efficacious. There is more; soon the pope came to be regarded as Christ's vicar on earth and infallible when he spoke "ex cathedra." What he said was law; he ruled and the people were to obey. Jesus hated this!

In contrast, Baptists believe that there is ". . . one mediator between God and men, the man Christ Jesus; . . ." (I Timothy 2:5). They believe that believers constitute a ". . . royal priesthood, . . ." (I Peter 2:9), and that they are invited to ". . . come boldly unto the throne of grace, that we may obtain mercy, and find grace to help in time of need" (Hebrews 4:16). This coming is directly through our one mediator, Jesus. He is the believer's Great High Priest. Baptists believe that pastors have no more right of access to God than individual believers have. With this teaching of Scripture, is it any wonder that our ancestors stood for an equal brotherhood of believers as far as access to God was concerned; and is it any wonder that they were soon on the receiving end of the hatred and opposition of those who had fallen for the error of the Nicolaitans?

With such plain Scripture to the contrary, we must wonder why anyone would succumb to such doctrine and practice as this. Perhaps a study of group dynamics will help us understand how this all came about.

THE FASTEST GUN IN THE WEST

In any group there will always be one who rises to the top as leader. Since a church is a group, this is true in them. Only one will rise to the absolute highest position; others will be in varying positions. Some of them will be near the top, some not so near; but there will never be two in a group that are equal in the highest degree of leadership.

Church history reveals that this is also true in groups of churches as well as in groups of people. As churches were established in different places, each of them had its own pastor or bishop. The word "bishop" is from the Greek word, *episcopos*; and its literal meaning is "overseer," or one who has the oversight of the church. His duties pertained only to the church he was over; and he had no authority, power, or responsibility over any other church. However, this was to change. Bishops of the larger churches came to be looked upon as being of a higher rank than those in the smaller churches. They began to be called *metropolitan bishops*. As time passed, some of the cities began to be looked upon as being more important than some of the others. Eventually, the church at Rome became the most important in the minds of many. According to tradition, Peter started this church and Paul had labored there. There is no biblical evidence that Peter was ever in Rome ; but according to the Catholics he was, and he had been given the keys to the kingdom. They say he, in turn, gave them to the bishops of Rome. The bishop of Rome came to be called *pope* from the Latin word, *papa* which means "father." He ruled over other churches as the head of the Roman Catholic Church and the hierarchy was begun, a hierarchy that gave the clergy rule over the laity. In this case, one had risen to the absolute highest position.

This principle of group dynamics also works in local churches. In such groups leaders emerge or are called, as in the case of pastors. Another principle of group dynamics comes into play here. When anyone occupies the highest position in a group, his leadership will be tested by some others in the group. Perhaps this is a play for power or for recognition. Human nature seems to demand that the one at the top be challenged. This was true in the old West; the "fastest gun" was the target of every young aspiring gunslinger. You never heard of anyone wanting to "shoot it out" with some old clodhopper who couldn't get his gun out of the holster without shooting himself in the foot. Many times people who have not learned the New Testament teaching of an equal brotherhood or of the priesthood of all believers test the leadership of the pastor and seem to want to shoot him out of the saddle. Many pastors seem to see their only hope of survival as shooting back. In this way, pastoral dictatorships sometimes come into being; and this can he a situation that comes very close to being the Nicolaitan rule over the people. Some pastors have never learned, practically, the lesson of the equality of all believers as it is taught in Scripture; nor have many members. Consequently, they have missed the benefits of the power that this biblical plan can harness as all believers work together in the church in order to carry out the task that God had given us to do.

THE PENDULUM SWINGS AGAIN

We must remember that pendulums also swing in the opposite direction and there is evidence in the book of The Revelation that it was going to do just that in this matter. The last of the seven churches was the one at Laodicea, and this word is also made up of two Greek words. They are laos, "the people" and dikao, "rule." Therefore the word can mean, "the rule of the people." The people in the age represented here are free from the rule of the clergy; but as is often the case, they went entirely too far and declared themselves independent of the rule of God also. To them, even the Bible was no longer authoritative. Notice the emphasis they now placed upon creature comforts and riches. "Because thou sayest, I am rich, and increased with goods, and have need of nothing; ..." (Revelation 3:17).

How did such a development as this come about? There is evidence that events surrounding the Reformation are greatly responsible. We stand amazed as we see how the Reformation fell far short of accomplishing what it might have done. Among other things, it was a protest against the ecclesiastical hierarchy of the Catholic Church; but it went to the opposite extreme and, being free from this absolute rule, was split by the abuse of its own liberty. As a result, Christendom was divided into many different denominations. So the desire of the people became the rule. If anyone did not like what was taught in one church, he had only to go to another. Sooner or later he would find one that agreed with him, thus making him the final authority or ruler in matters of religious faith and practice.

In the course of time, people began to realize that there were more "Indians than there were chiefs." Along with this came the realization that rulers ruled according to the consent of the ones governed. This idea even found its way into our Declaration of Independence:

> ... Governments are instituted among men, deriving their just powers from the consent of the governed, that whenever any form of government becomes destructive of these ends, it is the right of the people to alter or to abolish it, and to institute a new government, laying its foundation on such principles and organizing its powers in such form, as to them seem most likely to effect their safety and happiness ....

This is a hallowed document, and the sentiments expressed in it are correct, humanly speaking. However, no notice is taken of the fact that government is ordained of God and the powers of government are derived from Him (Romans 13: 1,2). Still, the governed must consent to be governed, either willingly or otherwise.

A good idea, taken to the extremes, becomes a bad idea. The government that grew out of the Declaration of Independence was to be based on law, and there is much evidence that it was to be derived from God's law. Problems came about when the different desires of each individual culminated in their demanding that their rights be guaranteed by law. It was then that the system broke down. It is impossible for us to demand our rights to have our desires fulfilled without turning away from God's law. Apply this principle to the church, and it is more obvious that peoples' turning to the fulfillment of their own desires will result in turning from God's will. The inevitable result is a Laodicean rule of the people.

The Baptist distinctive of an equal brotherhood probably came to light against the black backdrop of the Nicolaitan heresy; but this distinctive, improperly understood or taken to the extreme, can result in the Laodicean error. Our task in this work now becomes that of seeing how the Baptist distinctive of the priesthood of believers and of an equal brotherhood of believers fit between these two extremes. As we do this, we shall consider different forms of church government that came about and try to ascertain which is the most biblical. These systems of church governments will be positions that are taken somewhere between the Nicolaitan hierarchal rule of the clergy *over* the people and the Laodicean rule *of* the people.

Other than the two just mentioned, there are basically three kinds of church government. They are: (1) Congregational, (2) Episcopal, and (3) Presbyterian. We shall work from the last to the first in considering them. The congregational form will be seen to be the one that Baptists look upon as the one that best reflects their belief in soul liberty, an equal brotherhood, and the priesthood of believers.

PRESBYTERIAN

The word, Presbyterian, comes from the Greek word *presbuteros*, which means "elder." An elder was not an old man in his dotage; rather he was one who was not a novice, i.e., not one who was only recently converted to the Christian faith. In churches that have a Presbyterian form of government, these elders or presbyters are divided into two classes, teaching elders and ruling elders. The ruling elders do just that, rule, but not without some input from the members of the church. There is some evidence in the New Testament that churches had a plurality of elders; there is also reason to believe that this word did not designate a church office.

Let us look to the New Testament for a better understanding of elders. A careful study of Titus 1:5-9 indicates that the ones who were to serve as bishops, a term that I believe to be equivalent to the word, "pastor," were to be ordained from among the elders. Paul instructed Titus as follows, "For this cause left I thee in Crete, that thou shouldest ... ordain elders in every city ..." (v 5). However, when he listed the qualifications for those who were to be ordained, he gave qualifications for bishops. "For a bishop must be blameless, ..." (v 7). This does not mean that there were no men in these churches who were referred to as elders; but when one was ordained to have the oversight of a local church, he was called a bishop. All bishops were elders, but not all elders were bishops. There are indications that "bishop" refers to the office, while "elder" refers to the kind of man that filled that office.

EPISCOPAL

The Episcopal form of church government gets its name from the Greek word, episcopos, "oversight." This form of church government makes use of an overseer or bishop; but in this case, the bishop has the oversight of a number of churches instead of just one. Among the many things that he does for these churches is to appoint the one who is to serve as pastor for however long. Members of individual churches might influence his decision in this; but the final decision is, after all, his. This divides the body into unequal rank.

There is no doubt, the office of bishop is a biblical one; but in New Testament times, a bishop was the overseer of one local church. There is little, if any, evidence in Scripture that any man, or church, held any authority over any church other than his own. The only possible exception would be that apostolic authority that was wielded by men like Paul and Peter as they gave us the letters that help make up the New Testament canon of Scripture; but apostles have long since passed from the scene.

The fact that the sphere of a bishop's authority extended no further than his own local church does not mean that churches should not seek counsel from neighboring churches or from other pastors whose wisdom they respect. But in none of this should any order or rank exist that would, in any way, give any pastor or church authority over another church.

CONGREGATIONAL

A congregational form of government is a form in which all basic decisions are made by the majority vote of the members of the church. Thus, Baptists declare their independence, not only from any outside overlordship, but from any inside rule as well. Members may authorize committees or boards within the church to perform certain functions on their behalf. In such cases, these bodies could act after making certain decisions themselves without having the church vote on each detail; but they would be acting on the authority of the church. Baptists, historically, have used this form.

OF THE PEOPLE, FROM THE BIBLE

As a people who believe in the Bible as our only rule in matters of faith and practice, we must not use any particular form of government just because it fits our program. It must be biblical. Our task now is to see if there are New Testament examples of this being used in the early church and to see what is the scriptural position of those who assume places of responsibility. While there are no certain instructions in the New Testament concerning the form of government a New Testament church is to have, there are several examples that indicate that all the members were to be involved in the business transactions of the church.

First, we shall consider an incident that is recorded in the first chapter of Acts. It happened shortly before the day of Pentecost while the one hundred and twenty disciples were waiting in the upper room. Peter felt impelled to find a man to fill the place that had been left vacant by the death of Judas. In doing this, he stood in the midst of all of those who were gathered in the upper room and presented the matter to all of them. After he had made his presentation, explaining what he thought needed to be done, they gave forth their lots. While we do not know exactly what is meant by this, the language used does seem to indicate that each member had a part in it. So, in a primitive form at least, we have an example of each individual member of the body indicating, in some way or another, his personal preference as to one who would fill the vacancy. If this were all, it would hardly be enough, but there is more.

Acts 15 tells of the first church council. It was not a council in the sense of many churches coming together, but the church at Antioch sent delegates to the church at Jerusalem because of teachers who came from Jerusalem with whom they disagreed. It is possible that these teachers claimed to have been sent from the church there. The purpose of this council was to determine if the church at Jerusalem, and the apostles there, were in agreement with what they taught.

When the delegates from Antioch arrived "... *they were received of the church*, and of the apostles and elders, and they declared all things that God had done with them" (Acts 15:4). Some of the Pharisees which believed supplied the subject for debate by contending "... that it was needful to circumcise them, and to command them to keep the law of Moses" (v 5). Then we read, "And the apostles and elders came together for to consider of this matter" (v 6). This last statement sounds like only the apostles and elders made the final decision. However, after the matter had been thoroughly discussed, we read, "Then pleased it the apostles and elders *with the whole church,* to send chosen men . . ." (v 22). This is enough to show that the entire church was involved in the decision and in the action that followed. Study the entire passage carefully for yourself. This is an example of congregational government.

That the entire church was to act in matters of church discipline is shown in several places. In I Corinthians, chapter five, Paul tells them of a commonly reported sin in their midst. Then he proceeded to tell them what to do about it. They were to ". . . deliver such an one unto Satan . . ." (v 5). He explained further; they were to ". . . put away from among yourselves that wicked person" (v 13). This was to be done by the members of the church, not by someone who was over them. Paul said they were to take this action ". . . when ye are gathered together, . . ." (v 4). Evidently, this was to be done in one of their assemblies and was to be done by vote of the individual members. Later, in the second letter to the Corinthians, Paul told them to ". . . forgive him, and comfort him, lest perhaps such a one should be swallowed up with overmuch sorrow" (II Corinthians 2:7). This was evidently at a time after the man had repented; but the important thing is that he was to be forgiven by the members, not by some priest who could grant him absolution.

A further example of the part the members of the church are to play in its decisions and action is given in the instructions that Jesus gave for dealing with a brother who had trespassed against another. These instructions are recorded in Matthew 18:15-17. First, the offended one was to go to the one who had offended. If that did not produce results, he was to take one or two more with him; but if that failed, he was to tell the matter to the church and if he would not hear the church, he was to be looked upon as a heathen man and a publican. This was to be done by the church, not by some of the leaders only.

These examples seem to clearly indicate that each member was to have a definite part in the decisions and in the action that was taken by the church. This is indicative of a congregational form of church government. It should be noted, however, that the church, in its government, has only executive power, not legislative power. It can decide and state the way in which God's work will be done, i.e., how it will carry out what God has commanded, nothing more.

THE PROBLEM OF THE PASTOR'S POSITION

Within the congregational form of government there are different orders of responsibility, i.e., pastors and deacons. These are the only two biblical officers in a New Testament church and their authority or right to act comes from scriptural directives and they cannot go beyond that. Actually, their responsibility is to minister, biblically, to the members; and this makes them servants instead of overlords. However, there are times when pastors must speak with authority as they lead the flock of God.

It can readily be seen that such a form of government as this must be fine tuned; and even then, the problem of balance remains. Perhaps we can understand the equal brotherhood distinctive better in this form of government if we say, "We believe in an equal brotherhood of believers but not in a brotherhood of equal believers," i.e., not of believers having equal abilities, gifts, or responsibilities. They are equal before God, not before man. Someone must have the responsibility of leadership since everyone's responsibility is no one's responsibility. When anyone assumes this responsibility, he also assumes a different position and a certain authority; but this does not make him an overlord.

Let us look at the two biblical offices of a New Testament church, bishops (or pastors) and deacons. We need to see how they are to fit as leaders with a certain authority without doing violence to the Baptist distinctive of an equal brotherhood of believers.

First, deacons are viewed by many as a board that has authority much like the elders in a Presbyterian form of government. Consider two reasons that cause this not to be true: (1) the job description of deacons does not include authoritative action, and (2) the word "deacon" in the original language shows their position to be one of service, not authority. Understanding this will help balance whatever leadership authority they have with the equal brotherhood distinctive.

Consider first that the first deacons were chosen to act in a servile capacity (Acts 6:1-6). Notice especially, "Wherefore, brethren, look ye out among you seven men of honest report, full of the Holy Ghost and wisdom, whom we may appoint over this business" (v. 3). The business was that of seeing that the Grecian widows were not neglected in the daily ministration, i.e., of distribution of food. In other words, they were to serve tables (v. 2). However, their overall task was to serve in such a way as to relieve the preachers so they could "... give ourselves continually to prayer, and to the ministry of the word" (v. 4). Deacons were to take care of physical needs so the preachers could take care of spiritual needs. Scripturally, this can include many things, perhaps anything that will free the preacher to do what he is supposed to do. But this limits deacons to work that is servile, not authoritative.

In the second place, consider the meaning of the word, "deacon." In the Greek language it is "diakonos" and its basic meaning is "a servant of someone." It is very difficult to be someone's servant and to elevate yourself above that person to a place of authority. Therefore, the equal brotherhood distinctive is protected by proper application of these biblical truths.

Second, we will consider the office of pastor as it pertains to the equal brotherhood distinctive. Peter balances this well in his first epistle where he instructs elders who were acting in the role of bishops as they take the oversight of the flock.

The elders which are among you I exhort, who am also an elder, and a witness of the sufferings of Christ, and also a partaker of the glory that shall be revealed: Feed the flock of God which is among you, taking the oversight thereof, not by constraint, but willingly; not for filthy lucre, but of a ready mind; Neither as being lords over God's heritage, but being ensamples to the flock (I Peter 5:1-3).

More is involved in the pastor's position than this, however. He is not just one who serves. The Bible describes him as one who rules. The biblical qualification, found in I Timothy 3 states that he must be "one that ruleth well his own house, having his children in subjection with all gravity; (For if a man know not how to rule his own house, how shall he take care of the church of God?)." Further, three passages in Hebrews indicate that the pastor rules over believers. Consider the first two and notice that the context indicates rule in spiritual matters.

Remember them which have the rule over you, who have spoken unto you the word of God: Whose faith follow, considering the end of their conversation (Hebrews 13:7).

Obey them that have the rule over you, and submit yourselves: for they watch for your souls, as they that must give account, that they may do it with joy, and not with grief: for that is unprofitable for you (Hebrews 13:17).

However, a Baptist pastor is called by a vote of the people; and he can be dismissed in the same manner. Abuse of this fact could certainly prevent him from ruling effectively. How then, does he rule? Perhaps a better understanding of the meaning of pastoral rule, of his position, and of the proper value the people are to place on his ministry will help.

First, the word "rule" that we have just seen in the above passages comes from two different Greek words. The one found in Paul's letter to Timothy is from a word that means "to be over, to superintend, or to preside over." This meaning signifies good household management, but the fact that he is to have his children in subjection shows that he is to exert authority over them.

The word that is translated "rule" in the book of Hebrews is from a Greek word that means "to be a leader; to rule, command, to have authority over." This is a bit stronger than the meaning of the word "rule" that Paul used in Timothy. However, it is impossible to rule in either sense without exercising some authority. For a person to superintend or preside over a business or a body presupposes authority. To be a leader in the sense of ruling or commanding certainly requires it. But how does this fit in with the Baptist belief that a pastor is a part of an equal brotherhood of believers?

Consideration of the word, pastor, that is used of one who is in a leadership position in the church will help answer the above question. The word is used only once in the New Testament. The Greek word from which it comes is used many times, however; but all other times it is translated by the English word, "shepherd." That is exactly what a pastor is; it is also what a bishop is. A bishop oversees the sheep; so does a shepherd. A pastor leads the sheep; so does a shepherd. A shepherd leads the sheep in the path they should follow for their own good; it is the one that will lead them safely to the best pasture. He tells them where to lie down and when they are to do it. He also protects them by using his rod and his staff to keep them in line and away from dangerous places; and by the same means, he keeps them safe from the lion and bear. He does this for their good; but since he speaks authoritatively when he directs them in this, he becomes both their leader and their servant. Having understood this, we can begin to see the proper role of a pastor. He leads the people and he ministers to the people; and this helps balance his position in an equal brotherhood of believers. His understanding of this will help strengthen this balance. The people also have a responsibility in strengthening and maintaining this balance; they must be willing recipients of his ministry and leadership.

SCRIPTURE TO STRENGTHEN THIS ORDER

A passage of Scripture is given by the apostle Paul that will help members have the proper attitude toward their pastor. He wrote, "And we beseech you, brethren, to know them which labor among you, and are over you in the Lord, and admonish you; And to esteem them very highly in love for their work's sake . . ."(I Thessalonians 5:12-13). The important thing is the work, not the person. The work is that which each member of this equal brotherhood is trying to accomplish; and it is greater than anything or anyone that might act in such a way as to spoil this arrangement.

A further help to the people in giving the pastor his rightful place in leadership and responding to his leadership is a right understanding of who placed him in this position. The popular notion, as we have seen, is that the pastor is in his position because the church, congregationally, called him to it. Since they called him, they can uncall him if he does not please them. But as long as this notion prevails, the relationship between pastor and people will never prosper.

It is true that Baptists do call their pastors; but if the proper period of prayer and seeking God's will has been observed, he is called because he is God's man for that particular church. Paul, speaking to elders who were serving as bishops, said, "Take heed therefore unto yourselves, and to all the flock, over the which *the Holy Ghost hath made you overseers*, to feed the church of God, which he hath purchased with his own blood" (Acts 20:28). Since God has made a particular man the overseer of a particular flock, it is dangerous to remove such a person from the oversight of that flock without specific instructions from the One who placed him there. This will go a long way toward placing the pastor's position in the proper perspective.

ALL WHO MINISTER ARE NOT MINISTERS

One additional thought is necessary if the body of Christ that operates under a congregational form of government is to succeed; that is, each individual member is to minister. "Minister" is a word that can be used either as a verb or as a noun. The pastor is *the* minister; he is also *to* minister. Members are to have a ministry; and in fact, part of a pastor's task is to equip them for this ministry. This is seen clearly in the Expanded Translation by Kenneth Wuest. "He himself gave some . . . as pastors who are also teachers, for the equipping of the saints for ministering work with a view to the building up of the Body of Christ" (Ephesians 4:11-12 ET). So, although the responsibility of authoritative leadership rests on the shoulders of the pastor, the responsibility for the success of the work is shared by the members as they follow and do the work of the ministry. In this way, while all members may not have an office in the church, each one of them can have a ministry for Jesus.

This makes the work of a church possible and practical. Possible, because a handful of special people in a church are not enough to accomplish so vast a task. Practical, because this plan, properly used, sets a vast number of people to work under a God-ordained plan. Working this way, the church will no longer be a place for a few actors and many spectators; but it will be a place where each shares, through his own God-gifted ministry, in doing the job we have been given. This is congregational government at work. The people decide how they are going to do a task God has given them and then share in doing it!!!

CHAPTER IX
SAVED BY GRACE

God's grace is the theme of many of the songs we sing in our churches, and it is mentioned in many songs where it is not the central theme. Philip Doddridge wrote,

> *Grace ! 'tis a charming sound,*
> *Harmonious to the ear;*
> *Heav'n with the echo shall resound,*
> *And all the earth shall hear.*
>
> *Grace taught my wand'ring feet*
> *To tread the heav'nly road;*
> *And new supplies each hour I meet,*
> *While pressing on to God.*

Augustus Toplady added three more verses,

> *'Twas grace that wrote my name*
> *In life's eternal book;*
> *'Twas grace that gave me to the Lamb,*
> *Who all my sorrows took.*
>
> *Grace taught my soul to pray,*
> *And made mine eyes o'erflow;*
> *'Twas grace which kept me to this day,*
> *And will not let me go.*
>
> *O let thy grace inspire*
> *My soul with strength divine;*

*May all my pow'rs to Thee aspire,
And all my days be thine.*

Our sixth Baptist distinctive is that Baptists believe in salvation by grace, through faith, plus nothing and minus nothing. In considering this distinctive, we notice several things: (1) what grace is, (2) Bible teaching to show that salvation must be all of grace, (3) evidence that others do not teach salvation by grace alone, and (4) some ways in which Baptists inadvertently can come dangerously close to denying this distinctive in preaching and in practice. Perhaps no other part of this work is as important as this one, since to err in the way of salvation will affect our eternal destiny. We must be doctrinally correct here.

AMAZING GRACE (What Is It?)

It is impossible to see God's grace in its fullest form without exclaiming, "Amazing Grace." That being so, we do well to seek a full definition of this grace; and it has been variously defined. One of the simplest definitions is that grace is God's unmerited favor. Some, attempting to embellish this definition, have said, "Grace is God's unmerited favor bestowed upon undeserving men." Some have worded it a little differently and said, "Grace is God's favor, unmerited, unearned, and undeserved." All of these, however, say essentially the same thing. Using an acronym, some have said, "Grace is *G*od's *R*iches *A*t *C*hrist's *E*xpense."

While each of these definitions touches some aspect of grace, none of them goes far enough to show us the meaning of grace completely. It is true that grace is God's favor toward men; it is undeserved and unmerited. More than that, however, it is bestowed upon men who have done everything not to deserve it; and for that matter, they deserve just the opposite, God's wrath. Further, while each of these definitions does help us to understand the meaning of grace, we can get a much broader view from a study of Scripture that pertains to grace. After all, grace is a scriptural word; and we can expect Scripture to define it best.

One of the best known passages pertaining to grace is Ephesians, chapter two. Consider first, "For by grace are ye saved through faith; and that not of yourselves: it is the gift of God: Not of works, lest any man should boast" (v 8-9). Notice several things that are said about grace.

First, grace is not of ourselves as to its source, it is of God. Man, of himself, knows nothing of grace; and left to himself, man would never experience grace. Further, there is nothing in man that calls forth God's grace or that compelled or impelled Him to bestow grace on him. All of this motivation is found within the person of God and is activated by His attributes alone.

Second, grace provides salvation as a gift of, or from, God. Two things are implied in this. The first is that the recipient of a gift does not pay for it; this goes without saying. If he paid for all or part of it, it would not be a gift. The second implication is that the giver paid for the gift in full; and in this case it was at a great price, the blood of Jesus that was shed on the cross.

Third, salvation by grace is not of works on our part; however, it is by the work of Christ, which is a finished work. He has done all that is necessary; there is nothing we can add to it.

This is what grace does for those whom God saves; but we must go back a few verses and see what kind of people grace does this for. As you do, you will notice that there was no merit in any upon whom God bestowed His favor. Notice, they were

> ... dead in trespasses and sins: Wherein in time past ye walked according to the course of this world, according to the prince of the power of the air, the spirit that now worketh in the children of disobedience: Among whom also we all had our conversation in times past in the lusts of our flesh, fulfilling the desires of the flesh and

of the mind; and were by nature the children of wrath, even as others (Ephesians 2:1, 2).

But further, grace is superabundant. Notice how much farther it goes than that which is absolutely necessary. First, grace is that which quickens us, or gives us life (Ephesians 2:1-5). This is necessary. But still further, by grace God has ". . . raised us up together and made us sit together is heavenly places . . ." (Ephesians 2:6). There is more. It will take the ages to come for God to show us the exceeding riches of His grace (Ephesians 2:7). All this is done by grace which is of God, a gift, and not of works. No wonder Paul exclaimed a little later, "Now unto him that is able to do exceeding abundantly above all that we ask or think, . . . Unto him be glory in the church by Christ Jesus throughout all ages, . . ." (Ephesians 3:20, 21).

Consideration of at least one more verse of Scripture is necessary in order to establish that grace cannot include works, even in the smallest degree. Paul nailed this down for us when he wrote, "And if by grace, then it is no more of works: otherwise grace is no more grace . . ." (Romans 11:6).

From these things we have learned about grace we must conclude that saving grace must be pure grace with no mixture of works. However, since salvation is of grace through faith, does that not imply that man has some part in it? Wuest has an interesting comment on this.

> The words, "through faith" speak of the instrument or means whereby the sinner avails himself of this salvation which God offers him in pure grace. Expositors says: "Paul never says 'through the faith,' as if the faith were the ground or procuring cause of the salvation." Alford says: "It (the salvation) has been effected by grace and apprehended by faith" . . . .[1]

There are further indications in the Bible that even our faith, by which we apprehend salvation, is a gift of God. Paul wrote, "... For all men have not faith" (II Thessalonians 3:2). Therefore, if some do have faith it must be because God worked faith in them in some way. Faith, then, is a gift of God, and this shows further that salvation is all of grace and all of God.

SALVATION BY GRACE, A NECESSITY

So far we have considered Scripture that defines what grace is and what it does. This, in itself, indicates that salvation must be of grace; but there are many other passages of Scripture that indicate this truth, and there are biblical reasons for believing that men can only be saved by grace. There is no other way. If man tries to add works of his own, he negates God's grace. There are very good reasons why works of man cannot be added to God's grace. These reasons revolve around what man is and what he is not. Instead of looking at other Scripture that simply says salvation is by grace, we shall consider numerous passages that tell us why it must be this way. After doing this, we should be able to see clearly that salvation is by grace and that there is no other way.

Man Is Totally Depraved. Jesus must have been speaking of this when he told Nicodemus, "... Except a man be born again, he cannot see the kingdom of God" (John 3:3). Why must a man be born again? Because he was born wrong the first time. By birth, he is possessed of a corrupt, sinful nature that he is powerless to change. He is totally depraved. Total depravity has been defined in the following way:

> Total depravity means that sin has permeated every faculty of man's being just as a drop of poison would permeate every molecule of a glass of water. Sin has warped every faculty in man, and thus it taints his every act.[2]

Many verses of Scripture describe the various parts of man that are affected by this total depravity, thus showing that every part of man is tainted. Because of the extreme importance of this teaching, we will give the text of each of these verses.

(1) Man is depraved in mind: "And God saw that the wickedness of man was great in the earth, and that every imagination of the thoughts of his heart was only evil continually" (Genesis 6:5).

(2) Man is depraved in his heart: "The heart is deceitful above all things, and desperately wicked: who can know it?" (Jeremiah 17:9).

(3) Man is depraved in his affections: "And this is the condemnation, that light is come into the world, and men loved darkness rather than light, because their deeds were evil" (John 3:19).

(4) Man is depraved in his conscience: "Unto the pure all things are pure: but unto them that are defiled and unbelieving is nothing pure; but even their mind and conscience is defiled" (Titus 1:15).

(5) Man is depraved in speech: "The wicked are estranged from the womb: they go astray as soon as they be born, speaking lies" (Psalms 58:3).

(6) Man is depraved from head to foot: "From the sole of the foot even unto the head there is no soundness in it; but wounds, and bruises, and putrifying sores: they have not been closed, neither bound up, neither mollified with ointment" (Isaiah 1:6).

(7) Man is depraved from birth: "Behold, I was shapen in iniquity; and in sin did my mother conceive me" (Psalms 51:5).[3]

Certainly, this is enough to show that depravity has affected man's entire being. The result is that he can offer nothing that is acceptable to God because what he offered would come from a corrupted source. Just as a stream that comes from a polluted spring is polluted, works that originate in a corrupt person would also be corrupt. This could never be acceptable to God for our salvation.

But further, even if it were possible for a man to control himself to the extent that he never produced a bad work, the fact that he is corrupt would not be changed. A stream might be filtered to purify the water in it, but this would not purify the spring; and in man's case, the stream and the spring are one and the same. Man, who is corrupt, cannot stand before God regardless of how he might have made himself to appear. What he is must be changed, and only grace can do that.

Because of what man is by birth, he cannot be saved by works. Since he is basically unclean by nature, his works are odious to God. Notice Isaiah's pronouncement concerning this: "But we are all as an unclean thing, and all our righteousnesses are as filthy rags; and we all do fade as a leaf; and our iniquities, like the wind, have taken us away" (Isaiah 64:6). And Paul wrote, "Not by works of righteousness which we have done, but according to his mercy he saved us, . . ." (Titus 3:5). It had to be that way since unclean man could not offer anything acceptable to God who is ". . . of purer eyes than to behold evil, and canst not look on iniquity: . . ." (Habakkuk 1:13).

Further, man's total depravity prohibits him from earning salvation by keeping the law. First, it prevents him from keeping the law. "For what the law could not do, in that it was weak through the flesh, . . ." (Romans 8:3). Second, even if he were strong enough in the flesh to keep the law, that would not change what he is by nature. A fact that is not understood by most is that God is more interested in what we are than He is in what we do. Man's religiosity or piosity changes only outward appearances, not what man is by nature; and God is not interested in what we appear to be, only in what we are. These facts make salvation by grace a necessity; it is the only way.

Man Is Totally Helpless. When it comes to spiritual matters this is certainly true. He does not have the ability to do anything that will please God. His depravity renders him unwilling to submit to God, and his helplessness renders him unable to do this or anything else that will result in his salvation. We shall now consider a number of things that man is helpless to do apart from a special work of God. Notice that all of these things that man is helpless to do prevent him from doing anything for salvation and makes salvation by grace necessary.

First, he cannot see or enter into the kingdom of God. This was emphasized as Jesus stated the truth while speaking to Nicodemus who came to Him by night (John 3:3-5). Even if man could go to heaven in his natural state, it would not be heaven to him because his nature would render him unable to enjoy what he found there. Everything there would be against what he loved.

Second, natural man will not and cannot subject himself to the law of God. Paul wrote, "Because the carnal mind is enmity against God: for it is not subject to the law of God, neither indeed can be" (Romans 8:7). This, of course, refers to inward subjection, not outward conformity. However, one who will not and cannot subject himself to God's law will never conform to that law to any great degree.

Third, because of the fact he had just stated in verse seven Paul wrote, "So then they that are in the flesh cannot please God" (Romans 8:8).

Fourth, natural man cannot receive or know spiritual things. This inability is a serious hindrance to man ever having a right relationship with God. Notice the following proof of this inability.

> But the natural man receiveth not the things of the Spirit of God: for they are foolishness unto him: neither can he know them, because they are spiritually discerned (I Corinthians 2:14).

Fifth, natural man has absolutely no ability to withstand the devil. Paul exhorted Timothy to instruct those who oppose themselves, in order that "... they may recover themselves out of the snare of the devil, who are taken captive by him at his will" (II Timothy 2:26).

Sixth, he cannot cease from sin. Peter described some who had "... eyes full of adultery, and that cannot cease from sin; ..." (II Peter 2:14). This is shown in other Scripture and from experience; and again, even if man could discipline himself to cease from sin, the sin nature would still be present.

Seventh, man cannot come to Jesus of himself. This was stated by Jesus. "No man can come to me, except the Father which hath sent me draw him: and I will raise him up at the last day" (John 6:44). The last part of this statement shows that he was not speaking of a universal drawing; the one drawn will be raised up. A later verse shows the same truth. "And he said, Therefore said I unto you, that no man can come unto me, except it were given unto him of my Father" (John 6 :65). Man's inability to believe is also shown in the writings of Paul. "Wherefore I give you to understand, that no man ... can say that Jesus is the Lord, but by the Holy Ghost" (I Corinthians 12:3).

There is more, but this is enough to show man's absolute helplessness in spiritual matters. He is unable to do anything to commend himself to God. Therefore, salvation must be by grace; and as we have seen, by grace we are saved.

UNBELIEVING BELIEVERS

In the final analysis, the Baptists' troubles with others came about, largely, because of their belief in salvation by grace. Others claimed to believe in Jesus; but in one way or another, they demonstrated that they did not believe He could do the whole job. They had to help in some way; and of course, this nullifies salvation by grace.

Before looking in detail at some who did not believe that salvation was all of grace, consider several things in general that nullify this doctrine. Perhaps there are more, but we will look at only five. They are: (1) any belief that you or someone else except Jesus must do something for your salvation, (2) any belief that any act performed on your behalf, other than what Jesus has done, has salvific value, (3) any belief that some mediator other than Jesus is necessary for your salvation, (4) any belief that there is something you must do in order to keep yourself saved, and (5) a belief that you can be good enough to merit salvation. Belief in any of these indicates that a person is at least on shaky ground in the matter of salvation by grace and shows a need for further study of this important doctrine. Those with whom Baptists have differed held to some, or all, of these views; and this was manifested in many of their different doctrines and practices. In order to show this, we will refer briefly to some of the doctrines that have been discussed in previous chapters, doctrines against which Baptists historically have stood.

To begin with, infant baptism denies salvation by grace. It is an act performed by someone on behalf of another; and as we have noticed before, for anyone to believe that babies should be baptized, a belief that baptism has some salvatory value would have to prevail. This baptism is seen as a means of grace, but we have already seen that grace is not called forth by anything man can do. It is of God as to its source and application. Nothing man can do can cause it to be applied. If it could, salvation would not be of grace. Therefore, infant baptism is a denial of this doctrine. In this way Catholics have, through the centuries, denied this truth, as do all others who practice this ritual.

The Catholic doctrine of Transubstantiation denies salvation by grace. In the practice of this teaching, a priest is necessary to say the sacramental words that will turn the bread and wine into the body and blood of Jesus so another sacrifice can be made. This, in itself, implies several things. First, that the one sacrifice Jesus made on Calvary is not sufficient so others need to be made. Second, it is necessary for someone else, in this case a priest, to do something on your behalf to help in your salvation. Third, you must be there when it is done and partake of this sacrament. All in all, this means that there is something that you need to do and that someone else must do something for you for your salvation. This teaches against the sufficiency of the one sacrifice of Jesus and denies salvation by grace. Baptists stood against this ritual in the past and still stand today if they really understand salvation by grace. It was because of their refusal to take part in this that many of them suffered untold persecution in the past.

The Catholic doctrine of Purgatory denies salvation by grace. Remember, according to this teaching, purgatory is necessary because few are good enough to go directly to heaven or bad enough to deserve going directly to hell. Therefore, there must be some in-between place for those who don't really qualify for either place. They might not really be good enough for heaven because they did not do enough penance while on earth and so died with some sins unatoned for. Maybe they did not purchase enough indulgences while on earth; but have no fear, someone still on earth can purchase some for them or say prayers, light candles, have masses said for them, etc., in order to shorten the time the one in purgatory must spend there. This is salvation by works, not grace; and it also teaches that the sacrifice Jesus made was not sufficient to save completely, that there is something the seeking sinner can do to aid in his salvation, and that he can become good enough to merit salvation. According to Scripture, this is heresy; and one who loves the doctrine of Salvation by Grace will hate this teaching.

In the interest of brevity, we will discuss no more individual doctrines and practices of the Catholic Church. Suffice it to say that practically all of the sacraments of this church are something that must be done in order to aid in the process of salvation; and this being so, they deny that salvation is by grace, through faith,

We shall now turn to see ways in which many Protestants deny the doctrine of Salvation by Grace. We have already noticed that infant baptism is a denial of this doctrine because it is evidently done with the belief that it is somehow an aid to salvation. Another doctrine that denies grace is that of Baptismal Regeneration. The teaching inherent in this belief and practice is that it is necessary to be baptized in order to be saved. There are different degrees of emphasis in this. Some say only that baptism is a means of grace; but in so doing, they teach that it is necessary in order to convey God's grace to the believing sinner. In this they deny salvation by grace through faith. Others go farther, i.e., the Church of Christ, and declare that the salvation formula is "believe and be baptized." If one believes but is not baptized he is not saved. This certainly teaches that faith is not a sufficient channel of salvation, and the fact that something must be done teaches that salvation is not of grace since baptism is a work. Remember, if we add works to grace, grace is no more grace. Someone has remarked that to add water to the blood of Jesus dilutes it to the point that it cannot save.

It is not difficult to see that a belief that the initiatory rite of baptism is necessary to salvation would negate the doctrine of Salvation by Grace. However, at the opposite end of the spectrum is another belief that does the same thing. That belief is that a person can be saved by grace through faith but can then sin so as to be eternally lost. Those who claim to be saved in this way would, seemingly, be trusting Christ to save but not trusting Him to keep them saved. Their salvation would depend partly on what Jesus has done but partly on what they do. This would certainly deny that salvation is all of grace; and there is a big doubt, biblically, if such a belief can result in salvation.

Churches of the Reformation would certainly not be expected to hold any belief in Baptismal Regeneration and would be expected to hold to Salvation by Grace. However, there is evidence that this is not true and that, at least in the language of the Westminster Confession, some have retained certain vestiges of Catholicism in this matter. On the subject of baptism, the above mentioned confession states,

> Baptism is a sacrament of the New Testament ordained by Jesus Christ, not only for the solemn admission of the party baptized into the visible church, but also to be unto him a sign and a seal of the covenant of grace, of his ingrafting into Christ, of regeneration, of

remission of sins, and of his giving up unto God through Jesus Christ to walk in newness of life.

Hodge, a reformed theologian, reveals that he believes this statement means that baptism actually conveys grace to the one baptized. He wrote, "If they [baptism and communion] are 'seals' of the convenant, they must of course, as a legal form of investiture, actually convey the grace represented to those to whom it belongs."[4] This certainly causes us to suspect that they believe baptism has something to do with obtaining salvation, thus denying salvation by grace alone.

This suspicion is strengthened when we learn that the doctrine of a priesthood was retained by the framers of the Westminster Confession. Although it is not so called, there is evidence that this is true. This confession says, "There be only two sacraments . . . neither of which may be dispensed by any but a minister of the Word, lawfully ordained." Concerning this, Good says,

> . . . When this is connected with the position that these "sacraments" actually convey grace to the recipients, . . . it becomes apparent that for all practical purposes the "minister of the Word, lawfully ordained," *becomes a priest*. The grace-conveying "sacraments" are in his control[5] (emphasis is his).

This seems to be evidence enough to show that those who subscribe to the Westminster Confession all the way would have to admit to denying the doctrine of Salvation by Grace. Regardless of how sound they might be in other matters, this is a serious departure from the truth.

BAPTISTS BEWARE

How sad it would be if, after Baptists have stood for the doctrine of Salvation by Grace through the years, they were inadvertently to succumb to error in this matter. There is evidence that there is danger of doing just that. More and more Baptists are speaking of certain things that people are to do, or that they have done, in order to be saved; and they speak of them as if they were conditions of salvation. Further, many speak of these things as if they are depending on them for their salvation.

Before considering some of these things, let us make sure that we understand that the biblical way of salvation is through belief in Jesus. For instance, "... Believe on the Lord Jesus Christ, and thou shalt be saved, ..." (Acts 16:31). "He that believeth on the Son hath everlasting life: ..." (John 3:36). "Verily, verily, I say unto you, He that heareth my word, and believeth on him that sent me, hath everlasting life, and shall not come into condemnation; but is passed from death unto life" (John 5:24). Salvation is an internal transaction, not an external demonstration, notwithstanding the fact that there will be an external manifestation. Yet, some seem to be thinking more about external demonstrations as causes or conditions of salvation. Consider several of them.

First, some seem to think of "making a decision" as a condition of salvation; and this is encouraged by many evangelists. True, a decision is made, but it must be based upon belief; otherwise, a decision will be made to do something that cannot result in salvation. Further, belief or faith is the channel through which salvation is received, not the act of making a decision.

Second, some look upon the act of "walking the aisle" as being that which brings assurance, and possibly, salvation. Some years ago, a member of the church of which I was pastor was to have serious surgery. She spent the preceding weekend with her son, a professing Christian and a Baptist. Before attending church on Sunday he told her that he wanted her to "go forward" during the invitation. She reminded him that she was a believer, to which he replied that he knew that but he would feel better about her salvation if she "went forward" again. Such an attitude is dangerously close to denying salvation by grace.

Third, "praying the prayer" is a popular phrase. Recently, at the close of an evening service, a young man came on profession of faith. He said he believed and he had a repentant attitude. After the service another man questioned me about what he had done. I related how the young man had come and his seeming attitude, to which the man replied, "But did he pray the prayer?" Seemingly, in his mind, this was more of a condition of salvation than belief and repentance.

Fourth, I have been surprised to learn lately that many Baptists believe they are saved because they have asked Jesus to come into their heart. This is a salvation formula that is given many times when dealing with children about their salvation, and many of them can give no other reason for believing they are saved than that they have done that. However, this act is based upon faulty exegesis of a passage of Scripture, Revelation 3:20. It is altogether possible and probable that a person could verbally ask Jesus to come into his heart but not know who Jesus is or what He has done.

Now, we should realize that it is possible that all who are saved have done one or more of the above when they were converted; but these things were done as a result of a basic belief in Jesus. That belief is the channel through which salvation is received, not acts such as those we have discussed. It is when a person begins to look at acts such as we have considered as being the grounds of salvation that we are in danger of denying salvation by grace. Since there is evidence, or at least indication, that some are tending to go in that direction, we must make sure that we do not succumb to this error.

PREVENTIVE MEASURES

Briefly, there are some things we can do to help make sure we do not go astray in this matter. Consider them carefully.

First, an understanding of the doctrine of Salvation by Grace will help. This is especially true in regard to the biblical definition of grace, understanding what grace does and what kind of people it does it for, and of course, understanding man's basic makeup that makes salvation by grace the only way by which he could possibly be saved.

Second, knowing the way of salvation as revealed in Scripture is an absolute necessity. It is not enough to know some plan of salvation as revealed in a book. We should always check such as that by the final authority, the Bible. If we are not certain in this area we could well find ourselves giving others a false plan of salvation that could only result in disaster for them and cause us to be guilty of doctrinal error.

Our ancestors thought this doctrine was very important. Just how important it is to us will be determined by how careful we are to be correct in these matters.

BIBLIOGRAPHY

1. Wuest, Kenneth S., *Ephesians and Colossians in the Greek New Testament*. Grand Rapids, Michigan: Wm. B. Eerdmans Publishing Company, 1953. p 69
2. Simmons, Thomas Paul, *A Systematic Study of Bible Doctrine*. Daytona Beach, Florida: Associated Publishers, 1969. P 167
3. Ibid., pp 167,168. Summary
4. Hodge, A. A., D. D., *The Confession of Faith*. London: The Banner of Truth Trust, 1961 p 331
5. Good, Kenneth H., *God's Blueprint for a Church*. Des Plaines, Illinois: Regular Baptist Press, 1974. P 90

CHAPTER X
PRIMITIVE BAPTISTS

In Chapter I the fact that Baptists are an ancient people was established. Yet, their authenticity does not depend on being able to trace an unbroken succession of Baptist churches. It depends on their adherance to the Word of God. For that reason, the seventh distinctive that I have named has to do with Baptists maintaining the primitive order of the church. By this I mean that we are to look to the Scriptures, particularly those of the New Testament, for instruction in all of our beliefs and practices. We are not to adopt beliefs and practices that have evolved during the long history of the church just because they are taught by the church. Some of these came about because of unbelief and carnality. Admittedly, this distinctive is close to the first one we considered; but maintaining the primitive order has to do more with the practical side, putting into practice what we claim to believe. As we proceed, we will soon discover that this distinctive is very closely related to all the others just as the first is.

CARTS AND KINE

An Old Testament episode illustrates more fully what is meant by maintaining the primitive order. During the latter part of the period of the Judges, in the time of Eli, Israel lost the Ark of the Covenant to the Philistines during a battle. The Philistines jubilantly carried the Ark to the house of one of their gods, Dagon. However, on several successive mornings they found their god overthrown and broken. Soon, the people of their land were smitten with emerods, etc. They took counsel and determined that they must rid themselves of the Ark. Not knowing the proper way to transport it, they placed it on a new cart that was pulled by two milch cows that had young calves. Thus, it came to Beth

A PEOPLE FOR HIS NAME

Shemesh and was seen by the people there, on a new cart pulled by two cows.

A number of years later, David's kingdom was pretty well established and he sent to have the Ark brought up to Jerusalem. But the Israelites did not know the proper way to transport the Ark, and they evidently did not bother to go to the original source, the Law, to find how it should be done. Remembering that it had come to them on a new cart pulled by two cows, they placed it on a new cart pulled by two oxen. But, in doing this, they adopted a Philistine expedient, a method devised by heathen people who did not know Jehovah. Had they consulted the Law, they would have found that the Ark was to be carried by four men by means of staves that were placed through rings located at the four corners of the Ark.

As a result of transporting the Ark in the wrong way, when they came to the threshing floor of Nachon the oxen stumbled, and Uzzah put forth his hand to steady the Ark. This displeased God, who smote him and he died. All of this was because they had not gone back to the Scriptures to find the proper way to do God's work. Instead, they had used a method that had been handed down by unbelievers. They were quick to learn, however, and when three months had passed, David sent again to have the Ark brought up. We are told at that time, "And it was so, that *when they that bare the ark* of the Lord had gone six paces, he sacrificed oxen and fatlings" (II Samuel 6:13). Evidently, during this three months, they had searched the Book of the Law to find the primitive method of transporting the ark and now, men were transporting it according to the instructions God had given Moses originally. This time the Ark reached Jerusalem safely, and therein is the saying fulfilled, "If all else fails, read the instructions." Go back to the basic message of God's Word.

UNWILLING REFORMERS

In an earlier chapter we noticed that, at first, the Anabaptist joined with the Reformers in the work of the Reformation. However, they soon discovered that the Reformers were not willing to go far enough and break completely with the Catholic Church. Instead, they retained quite a few of their doctrines and practices. In many doctrines in which they did depart from the Catholic Church, their departure was more of a compromise than a complete break. Repeatedly, they refused to return to the primitive order of the church. They just were not willing to go back to the Bible and follow that alone as their rule of faith and practice. Consider several examples of this.

At first, Martin Luther evidently did not intend to break with the Catholic Church. Instead, he wanted to reform it and rid it of many things that he saw as abuses. However, much of the form and philosophy of the church would be retained; and its goals would still be the same, i.e., a universal church ruling to the uttermost part of the earth as the Kingdom of God. Remember, this Church used coercion to propagate and perpetuate this kingdom; and much of its form, philosophy, and doctrine was based on tradition, not on God's Word.

Perhaps the main thing that moved Luther to speak out was the Catholic practice of selling indulgences. Indulgences could be purchased from the Catholic Church and could be used instead of doing penance. One who had a loved one in purgatory could purchase indulgences for that person and shorten the time he had to spend there. I suppose they could also be purchased in advance in order to shorten, or perhaps eliminate, the time a person was going to have to spend in purgatory. This is still a part of the practice of the Catholic Church today. It is interesting that, when Luther nailed his ninety-five theses to the church door at Wittenberg, he did not attack indulgences as such; instead, he addressed the abuses that had come to be associated with them. Had he searched the New Testament and been willing to return to the primitive order that is found there, he would have been forced to say that the basic wrong of indulgences is not the abuses but the indulgences themselves. Here, we get our first clue that, although Luther's watchword was "Sola Scriptura" and although he did come to the biblical doctrine of Justification by Faith, he was not going to be willing to forsake tradition altogether and look to the Scriptures as his only guide. He failed in many ways to go back to the New Testament for the primitive order of the church.

This hesitancy to go all the way is shown further in that, while Luther was in exile at Wartburg Castle, some of his followers began to attempt many radical changes. Luther came out of exile, returned to Wittenberg, and stopped these radical Reformers. Some historians credit him with wisdom for doing this; and perhaps, it was wise in the short run. However, in the long run, it seems that more would have been accomplished in reforming the church if he had been willing to follow the teaching of Scripture completely.

We have already seen that Luther did not believe that infant baptism could be proved from Scripture. Yet, he was not willing to forsake tradition. He felt that to depart from doing a thing that had been practiced for so long a time would be too radical, so he retained the practice.

Luther did depart a great deal from the Catholic doctrine of Transubstantiation, but he stopped short of teaching that the Lord's Supper is only a memorial that shows, symbolically, the body and blood of Jesus. Luther did not believe that the bread and wine actually become the body and blood of Jesus, but he did believe that His body is present in the Supper. John Calvin went a step further, but still not far enough, when he taught that Christ is actually present in the bread and wine, not bodily but spiritually; and by faith, those taking the Supper partake of Him.

This is in no way an attempt to discredit Luther. He was a great man and was greatly used in breaking the dominion of the Roman Catholic Church. In fact, he stood for some of the truths for which the Anabaptists stood, although certainly not all of them. Luther rejected the papacy. The distinction between the clergy and laity was broken, and he taught that all believers are priests. He believed in only two sacraments, Baptism and the Lord's Supper. He also taught that these ordinances were not essential to salvation. He rejected prayers to the saints and to Mary as well as many of the other trappings of the Catholic Church. However, while he changed many things about the church, he did not do away with anything that was not directly forbidden in the Bible, although many of these things had evolved from tradition and had no biblical basis. The Reformation could have been much more complete if he had used the New Testament as a model of what a New Testament church should be. Then, and only then, would there have been thorough Reformation.

DIFFICULTIES OF REFORMATION

While pointing out the places in which Luther failed in completely reforming the church, we can also sympathize with him. It is very difficult to effect complete reformation of any organization, especially if that organization has strayed very far from what it should be. This was certainly the case with the Catholic Church when he attempted to reform it. It is easier to continue doing what you have been doing, that to which you have become accustomed and with which you are comfortable. There is a feeling of security in sameness. This is true even if the thing we are doing is wrong. When it has become traditional, we tend to stop thinking in terms of right or wrong. We reason that if it is tradition it must be all right. In fact, it is sometimes hard to see that anything else could be right.

By way of illustrating this, consider why it is that the services of our churches are almost always structured so that the people are arranged in rows, one behind the other, with the preacher and the choir at the front facing them. Some time ago, a church was started. The place of meeting was to be in the dining room and living room of a private home. Sufficient chairs were secured and then placed row after row with a place for the piano and the preacher at the front. Why? Because this is the way we do it. However, there is a good chance that early church services which were held in private homes were structured so that the believers faced one another. Now, there is nothing wrong with either of these arrangements, biblically. Row after row is possibly the best for preaching, although not for fellowship since it is hard to fellowship with the back of the next person's head. Recently some writers have recommended the latter arrangement but are quick to admit that it would cause a good bit of objection.

Now, the point of all this is not that it is biblically wrong to sit in rows for the church service, but that it would be difficult to change and do it any other way. Why? Simply because we have become accustomed to doing it this way; it is tradition! So we who reject tradition as authoritative sometimes bow before it in matters of practice. This principle points out the need consciously to seek to find the Bible way for everything we do.

Having said this, let me hasten to say that many times the Bible does not prescribe the way we are to do things. We are just told to do them. It does not tell us to sit in rows or to sit facing one another. As a matter of right and wrong it does not matter. In effecting a certain goal it might. In the matter of missions we have no instructions as to how we are to go to the uttermost part of the earth. We are just told to go. The Great Commission does not say whether to go by ox cart or by jet liner. Had it done so, a primitive means of transportation would, no doubt, have been prescribed. Exegetes would certainly have had room to ponder if mention had been made of jet liners. However, so that the Bible could continue to be timeless as well as timely, the method of travel was omitted. It makes no difference how a missionary gets to the field. We have great freedom in the method we use when none is prescribed. It is important that missionaries get to the field, and the message they preach is of the utmost importance. Here we have no latitude; we are bound by Scripture as to the content of our message as we preach, whether at home or in the regions beyond. We do need to be certain that, whether the way we do a thing is prescribed in Scripture or not, the thing we are doing is scriptural.

BACK TO SQUARE ONE

Baptists are a people of the Book; they also place a great deal of importance on doctrine. Seemingly, these two would go together. Yet, frequently when Baptists are asked why they believe what they believe, their attitude is, "Because that is what Baptists believe." However, that is not good enough. Some who have called themselves Baptists in the past have erred grievously in doctrinal matters. To have believed something just because they believed it would have resulted in grave doctrinal error. Again, the Bible is the only safe guide. We must always be able to say, "I believe because it is taught in Scripture."

Further, what Baptists believe today might not be what they have believed in the past. For instance, most present-day Baptists do not put much emphasis on the Doctrines of Grace, commonly called Calvinism. This teaching has to do with the decrees of God, election, effectual call, etc. However, it is not possible to study the history of Baptists, especially the history of their doctrine, without taking note of the fact that, historically, they have held this doctrine. This is clearly shown by their confessions of faith. The London Confession which was adopted in 1689 was patterned after the Westminster Confession, which was strongly Calvinistic. The Philadelphia Confession, adopted in 1742, was very similar. The New Hampshire Confession, adopted in 1833, was the result of a controversy with the Free Will Baptists who were Arminian in theology. Although this confession might be seen as a compromise due to this controversy, it still retains a theology of moderate Calvinism. In addition to this, many of the men who founded the first Baptist seminaries in our land were quite Calvinistic. But this alone, does not make it right to hold this belief.

Still futher, Calvinism is usually identified by its five points; but these were not formulated by Calvin. They came about as an answer to the five articles of Arminianism; and they were stated in their present form by the Synod of Dort in 1618-19, more than fifty years after

Calvin's death. They do consist of things that Calvin taught and, perhaps, popularized; so the term "Calvinism" has become a name to identify those who subscribe to all, or most, of the five points. However, some insist that the origin of this teaching was not with Calvin but with Augustine, since he also taught many of these same things many years before. Perhaps Calvin followed Augustine. Any doctrine, however, must be held because it finds its origin in the Scriptures, not because it was taught by some man or men in the past. These who hold this doctrinal system do base it upon the teaching of the Bible; but in spite of this, some seem to have a tendency to appeal to these men about as much as they do to the Scriptures.

We need to be very careful in identifying with those in the past without knowing the biblical basis of their belief. It is generally unwise to apply their brand indiscriminately. Actually, it is inconceivable that any Baptist would use the Calvinistic handle for any other reason than to identify himself with the Doctrines of Grace. Although Calvin was used greatly in this area, we certainly could not identify with him in other things. He was a Pedobaptist. He was instrumental in the burning of Servetus at the stake, thus showing a belief in coercionism which could only be understood as pointing to a belief in a State-Church in spite of the fact that he denied the state any power over the church. These are things that we have seen to be wrong, things that caused our predecessors much suffering. Calvin's actions fly in the face of our distinctives. Therefore, in identifying with any man, it would be wise to explain what part we accept. Better still, base all doctrine on Scripture.

The danger of building on another's foundation is possibly shown further in a study of Calvin's millennial views. He dismissed pre-millennialism by saying, "Their fiction is too puerile to deserve refutation." It sounds as if he might have been reading Augustine at that time; for Augustine had said of pre-millennialism, "It were a tedious process to refute these opinions point by point." Could it be, as these statements seem to indicate, that Calvin simply accepted Augustine's opinion of pre-millennialism and that neither of them ever really attempted to refute these views. Perhaps, without considering these views, Augustine went ahead to develop his theory of the millennium, a theory based on unsound principles of Bible interpretation that became the foundation for the Catholic dogma of a universal church ruling absolutely over the earth. If this is so, an irrefutable case is made for going back to the Bible, the primitive source.

The danger of appealing too much to the teaching of some man who wrote since the completion of Scripture can be seen if we realize that men make mistakes. Sometimes they are correct in one area but dead wrong in others. They can be right about the Doctrines of Grace, but absolutely wrong in matters of baptizing infants, of church and state, etc. When we study the teachings of others, we must be especially careful to be sure that Scripture references say what they claim they say. Many teachers, past and present, display an uncanny ability to make it appear that their teaching has the backing of the Bible. Upon close scrutiny, however, it is often found that their views are not supported by Scripture. Only a Spirit-led study of the original source for the primitive order will reveal this; and we must use Spirit-given discernment as we consider what others teach. This is true regardless of whether the system we are considering is that of Calvinism, Covenant Theology, Dispensationalism, British Israelism, Millennialism, or whatever. These must be tested in the crucible of God's Word. This is what we mean by going to Scripture for the primitive order of faith and practice.

NEW THINGS IN THE OLD

Standing for the primitive order of the church does not mean that we must not use new things, new methods, or new ideas. Some having erred here have allowed themselves to stagnate; and they have become an oddity, attracting attention to themselves rather than pointing to Jesus whom they claim to serve. A thing is not bad just because it is

A PEOPLE FOR HIS NAME

new, nor is it good just because it is old. The order revealed in the New Testament must be our final guide. Paul wrote, "Prove all things; hold fast that which is good" (I Thessalonians 5:21). Alexander Pope wrote, "Be not the first by whom the new is tried, nor yet the last to lay the old aside." The Scriptures must be our guide in deciding.

Standing for the primitive order of the church does not mean that we cannot discover new truth. This is certainly true concerning individuals who are growing in the knowledge of His Word. I believe it is also true of truth in general. To deny this would mean that all truth has been gleaned from God's Word and that there is nothing more to discover. Joseph Parker said, "When the last word has been said about the Bible it will no longer be the Word of God." The Bible does contain truth that, at the time of writing, was to be sealed until a certain time.

Consider first, after Daniel had written most of his prophecy he was told to ". . . shut up the words, and seal the book, even to the time of the end: . . ." (Daniel 12:4). There are, no doubt, many different ideas as to when the "time of the end" will be. However, it is evident that there was some message in this book, some truth that could not be known until that time. If this is not true, what was the purpose of sealing the book? If this is true, and the "time of the end" has not come yet, there is still truth to be revealed.

Consider further, that in spite of much guessing on the part of students of prophecy, the identity of the beast out of the sea in Revelation, chapter thirteen, is still not known. We can't identify him today. What, then, is the purpose of the description of this beast and of his identifying mark? Why don't we know who he is? First, we do not need to know because we are not confronted by him. His identity is not needed now. Evidently, his identity will be made known to those saints who are living when he is revealed. In this case, truth is concealed, but it will be revealed in the future to those who need it.

Consider also that according to James Orr in *The Progress of Dogma*, the order in which different doctrines have been considered and developed has corresponded chronologically with the general order that is followed in most systematic theologies, i.e., apologetics, theology proper, anthropology, Christology, soteriology, and after the Reformation, eschatology. This would explain why some truth was discovered relatively late, and that some may still be discovered.

When a claim is made that new truth is discovered, however, we must check it out by God's Word. It must not be merely some system of doctrine that is just an outgrowth of the reasoning of the mind of man and that has no biblical basis. Further, we must remember that when new truth is discovered it will never contradict old truth. Truth is always in harmony with truth.

THE RESULT OF THIS STAND

Because of their belief in the Bible as their only authoritative rule in faith and practice, and because they constantly put this principle into practice, those who preceded us became a thorn in the flesh to those in the established church. They were a constant reminder to them that they were not on biblical ground in what they were doing. They were a constant threat to the progress and success of the State-Church. Their preaching of salvation by grace was a constant source of condemnation to those who sought to establish salvation by any other method. As a result they were always under the derision of those who were opposed by them.

Because they carried the gospel to the people, they received the name, "ale house preacher." They were accused of disturbing the peace at times because, the authorities said, "You can't meet one of them on the street without having them ram a text of Scripture down your throat." Because they had to resort to secret places for worship, they were called "hedge-row preachers." Their practice of rebaptizing brought forth the derisive designation of "Anabaptists." Because they insisted on immersion as the only means of baptism, they were called by the time-honored name, "Baptists."

But, there is more. They also won for themselves a place in history as thorough reformers simply because they insisted on going all the way back to Scripture in what they did. If a thing was not biblical, they refused it. If it was, they insisted on it. What a simple formula for knowing God's will! In the past century, John Quincy Adams wrote a book entitled, *Baptists the only Thorough Religious Reformers*. Needless to say, he believed that they were the only ones who were willing and able to bring about the reform that was needed. However, they were not reformers in the sense of the others because they were just continuing to do what they had been doing.

Because of our rich heritage, Baptist churches today are relatively simple in their organization. They still claim to be independent, even in the most rigidly organized conventions. Perhaps this, along with their practice of looking to the Bible as their authority, is the reason that many preachers who have been educated in doctrinally unsound seminaries have remained relatively sound. Most Baptists are not overly liturgical. Their order of service is fairly simple, and their chief concern still seems to be preaching the gospel, teaching the Word, baptizing believers scripturally, and practicing the observance of all things that we are told in God's Word. Their work is centered around the task of the local church, not around building a kingdom that will reach and control the world. Their motive in doing this is that God might be glorified. May we ever continue in this way!!!

-END-